Which Doctor?

An Australian Woman's Journey to Health and Wellbeing

DR NERIDA JAMES

Naturopathic Physician

Homeopath

ND; DC; Dip Irid; Cert Hom.

A special thank you to my daughter Afrika as the artist who painted the beautiful image on the front cover of the book as well as the flowers inside the pages.

You are a gift to my life. Thank you for sharing your gift for this book.

Dedication

Utmost in my heart is Dr. Nelly Laws who was the principal of the Laws College of Naturopathy and Chiropractic, who accepted me. Without her school and its knowledge, I would never have reached the know-how that I now impart to you, the reader.

I want to especially dedicate this book to my daughters, who put up with years of their mother's work, training, conferences, and patients, who were at times in our home and often kept me late getting home to them both. Also, to their husbands and my five adorable grandbabies, who make my life a joy.

I also dedicate this book to you, the reader, for you are in search of answers and herein, I truly hope you find a crack in the door of such an answer.

I would be remiss in not also dedicating this book to my life partner, for he has been my rock and go-to for all technical issues I have faced in putting this book together.

Foreword

*W*hich Doctor?, by Dr Nerida James, gives excellent examples and supporting evidence of effective outcomes where natural therapies have been successful in bringing about desired results, and acknowledges that traditional and complementary medicines can work together.

The book makes a highly valuable contribution to community wellbeing with, among other things, the seemingly simple message – drink more pure water, maintain a healthy diet with fresh vegetables, and emphasises the importance of regular exercise to take control of your wellbeing. It reinforces the idea that this is one of the best ways to establish a healthy body to give strength to its immune system.

As the former Member of Parliament for Springvale, and as the current Chairperson of the Ethnic Communities Council of Victoria, which is the peak organisation representing 200 ethno-specific organisations in this state, I have worked extensively, over many years, in numerous drug and health related environments, as well as sitting on many committees at both the Victorian Parliamentary as well as the local community level.

Some of these roles have included being a member of the Victorian Parliamentary Alternative Medicine inquiry where I developed links with the complementary medicine community and was also the Chairperson of the Springvale Community Health Centre Board of Management, running needle exchange and youth programs such as the Shack.

I have known Dr James for more than 30 years, have developed and maintained regular communication with her during that time, and have visited several programs and initiatives she has been involved in.

It has been a pleasure working with Nerida over this long period of time, and I welcome her contribution with this outstanding publication. It gives a real insight into how success can occur when you are determined, as she says, to "take back your power".

Eddie Micallef

Contents

Introduction 1

Natural Medicine: My Personal Story 6

Chapter 1 — Take Your Power Back for
                Lasting Wellness 36

Chapter 2 — My Philosophy for Lasting Wellness 42

Chapter 3 — Iridology - Iris Diagnosis, A Dying Art 54

Chapter 4 — Alternatives To Medicating Your Child 76

Chapter 5 — Hormone Balance 106

Chapter 6 — Cancer: A Foot in Both Camps 135

Chapter 7 — Anxiety, Depression, Insomnia –
                Alternatives to Medicating Yourself 155

Chapter 8 — Allergies & The Immune System –
                Autoimmune Diseases 178

Chapter 9 — Energy Medicine: It Takes All Kinds 197

Chapter 10 — Stand-Out Success Stories 206

Conclusion 218

Success Stories 221

Herbal Tonics – Nerida's Elixirs 228

Resources 242

Acknowledgements 317

About The Author 319

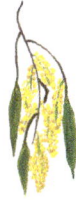

Introduction

Which Doctor do I go to now?

How many times have people asked themselves that question?

"I have a mild cold or cough and need time off work. Where can I get some general advice?"

Your local GP or your local Naturopath can give you that advice: both can give you a work certificate for time off to recover and recommend a few simple tips to help you or a loved one through that illness. Perhaps it may be a bladder infection, an ear infection, the flu, or some other viral infection.

But *which doctor* do you choose?

What if you have a more serious condition? You have severe back pain; you have debilitating migraines; you haven't had a menstrual cycle for several months; you're worried about your health in general and just want a check-up.

Maybe your asthma has flared up and your inhaler just isn't working anymore, nor is your preventer, and you are still struggling to breathe?

Maybe you have an autoimmune disease and on immunosuppressant drugs and the cortisones scare the hell out of you or you just don't want to stay on these medications long-term and you're struggling with the side-effects...*which doctor* do you consult? You have already been to three GPs, two specialists, and you still don't have an answer...*which doctor* do you see now?

These and many more scenarios have been asked over and over in the last 100+ years by many seeking help, knowledge, understanding, and solutions for their health.

If you are one of these people, this book could well be your answer.

I wanted to write this book to leave a legacy after a lifetime in practice as a naturopathic physician, homeopath, remedial massage therapist, NAET practitioner, and chiropractor. I wanted to share with as many people as possible that there are solutions to pain, physical and emotional, without the use of pharmaceutical drugs that create so many side-effects. At times, these chemicals do not help at all; nor does the use of surgery, which should be our last resort and not our first choice.

I have been, and still remain, an extensive collaborator with both medical and allied health professionals, and I believe the medicine of the future is the coming together of both allopathic (medical) and naturopathic care. Using both modalities and other techniques such as acupuncture, chiropractic, osteopathy, and homeopathy will ensure working in collaboration with medical assistance to achieve the best possible outcomes for each person seeking help.

There are so many herbal tinctures, homeopathic medicines, nutritional supplements, as well as physical therapies that can bring a suffering person and, at times, a dying person back from the brink to achieve health and wellbeing once again.

All of the possibilities, all of the techniques available, *should* be well-known by those searching both for answers and solutions to life's sufferings, not to mention the vast importance of counselling, spiritual solace, and connection, which is being pushed aside in this day and age for a quick-fix pill.

This book includes subjects that I see patients coming into the clinic with on a daily basis that are challenged by:

- Conditions they are frustrated with due to the lack of guidance not given to them by their specialist or GP;

- Patients who don't feel educated or empowered in any way by our current mainstream medicine approach towards wellness;
- Patients that lack any form of accurate diagnosis.

This shortfall of poor diagnostic techniques is largely due to the reliance on blood testing as the be all and end all for the local GP. But these methods of testing are limited and due to homeostasis (the body's ability to keep our blood chemistry balanced at all times), means having only the blood work approach is a very narrow view of whole-body health.

Looking at your tongue, your fingernails, and inside your eyelids while also taking down a thorough case history of your habits and lifestyle is not possible anymore due to the time restraints put on the family GP. How often does he or she even check your blood pressure during an appointment these days? Once upon a time, it was done in each and every visit.

Within this book, I hope to guide you through some important topics, including:

- Allergies and the immune system
- Hormone balance for teens, young women, older women, and men

- Cancer and many available treatments that are not spoken of in mainstream medicine

- Depression, anxiety, and insomnia, as well as all the alternatives available to assist a person greatly with these symptoms without the use of drugs or shock treatments that are still regularly administered even now

- Caring for your child's health without the use of harsh drugs and chemicals, or even surgery – which should be a last resort

- And finally, natural medicines: what is possible and the miracles I have witnessed

I have also included many of the herbal formulas I developed over the years that are highly effective. You can find these at the end of the book under Resources for you to use and perhaps source from your integrative GP, your herbalist, or your Naturopath. This book is to expand your knowledge and your practitioner's knowledge of what is truly available to you for your healthcare.

My hope for you as the reader, being a person who is seeking answers and solutions, is that you will use this book as reference material and a guide to carry you forward on the journey of creating and sustaining the best possible health and wellbeing throughout your life.

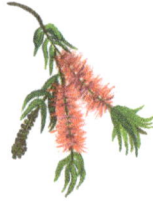

Natural Medicine:
My Personal Story

I was born in the state of New South Wales in Australia. Soon after I was born, I suffered chronic diarrhoea for 18 months, until a paediatrician 300 miles away finally diagnosed me with celiac disease. I was taken off wheat and gluten, and I finally became well until I turned three years old.

At this age, I went back onto white bread and lots of dairy milk. Then, I started having chronic tonsillitis with repeated courses of antibiotics. At five years old, I had such rotting tonsils that they fell apart in the surgeon's hands. After this, chronic bronchitis settled in and, again, I was given repeated courses of antibiotics.

At the age of 10 years old, I watched my baby brother nearly die from whooping cough, which he had contracted from receiving the vaccine itself. For weeks, I helped my mother to care for him by staying up late and even through the night to allow her to get some sleep. You see, someone had to be there pick my brother up if he started coughing. If you left him lying down, he would go blue and start choking trying to get his breath. It was then, as a 10-year-old, that I thought to myself that if this is what happens to a baby when he gets vaccinated, I am never doing this to my children!

On my 11th birthday, I started menstruating at a school camp without knowing what was happening in my body. I went rushing to the girl who was looking after our dormitory and said in great distress, "You need to take me to the hospital. I'm bleeding to death." After cleaning me up, she sat me down and explained fertility, a woman's hormonal cycle, and the normalcy of a monthly bleed. In those times, it seems that mothers didn't talk to their daughters about menstrual cycles or fertility. I went home feeling so mad at my mother for never even once mentioning this would happen to me as a natural part of growing up and becoming a woman.

At this same time, my acne set in. It was mortifying. No number of pharmacy acne lotions did anything to alleviate my facial condition. No number of trips to the doctor, where I was often told that I would grow out of it, helped either.

When I was 13 going on 14 years old, my parents separated. This was devastating for me, not just because of the separation, but also because of the pain of living at home with my dad who would cry at night, suffering the weight of the loss. I recall one night that he had his head on my lap. I was consoling him, telling him it would be all right and patting his back in reassurance. Neither parent really wanted me to live with them, so it was decided that I would go to a boarding school.

I think this was largely due to me being an angry teenager who also needed to go to high school, but did it *have* to be so far away from the farm I was raised on and where I had my horse that I needed to ride every day? I was used to living on a farm of 1200 acres, riding my horse, helping Dad round up cattle or sheep at shearing time, and being the roustabout. I also knew about wool classing.

It was only once I was in the institution that I discovered to my horror that I was only allowed out twice a year. This was after being told that I would be able to go home every weekend. I was boarded in a room with five other girls that had bars on the windows. I felt betrayed, to say the least. I was imprisoned for being the child of my parents and taken away from the country life I loved so much, as well as away from my mum, dad, brother, and sister. Needless to say, an institutional boarding school was a rude awakening to another side of life, one that had mean and nasty girls who swore and regularly took drugs – something very foreign to me.

After two months at this boarding school and not seeing any family or my horse, I decided I was going to run away. One night, I scrounged up a whole $8.00 and, in between nightly security rounds, I loosened the bars on one of the windows, snuck passed the adult in charge of our dorm, and escaped.

I hitchhiked from the country boarding school to Sydney, 300 miles away. I was well cared for as I hid with those whom I came across on my journey to what I felt was freedom. I was taken in by young people also finding their way in the world. They were kind to me and fed me, gave me a bed to sleep on until I found somewhere more permanent.

Then the *Sydney Morning Herald* published a photo of me with the headline "Missing Country Girl Being Hidden by Junkies" on page 3. I was never hidden by junkies. In the article, it said that I was being looked after by prostitutes, which also never happened. But this is typical of the media and the news sensationalising any story to make it seem more devastating.

At that point, I had just gotten a job as a sales girl in a local retail store in a Sydney suburb and realised that I would now be more easily recognised as the missing country girl. So, I turned myself in to the Paddington police station in Sydney. I was then taken back to the country area I came from, only to be fostered out to my dad's twin brother and his wife. I finished 4th form (year 10 now) while living with them and their children.

I decided that despite achieving five straight A's in my exams, I would learn more from life than further schooling. I could not see the use of memorising dates of things that happened centuries ago or remembering the names of people long since dead or even reading some book written by a person that knew nothing about the world in which we live today. There was nothing practical that I could learn at school after reading, writing, and arithmetic that was going to give me any help to survive alone in this crazy world. So, I decided to leave school and go out and explore the world and find out what it was that I wanted from life.

I was 14 years old and determined to make my own way in the world without being part of the challenging divorce that my parents were going through. My little brother and sister were in the care of my mother and my grandmother, whom I had always gotten along well with. Grandma Cobb taught me to paint with oil paint and acrylics, which I still enjoy to this day.

I kept my own counsel and decided that if I was going to find my purpose in life, if I was going to be happy, I could do so much more easily without all the drama of my family and the institution called high school.

So, I left school, left home, and went to live in Sydney.

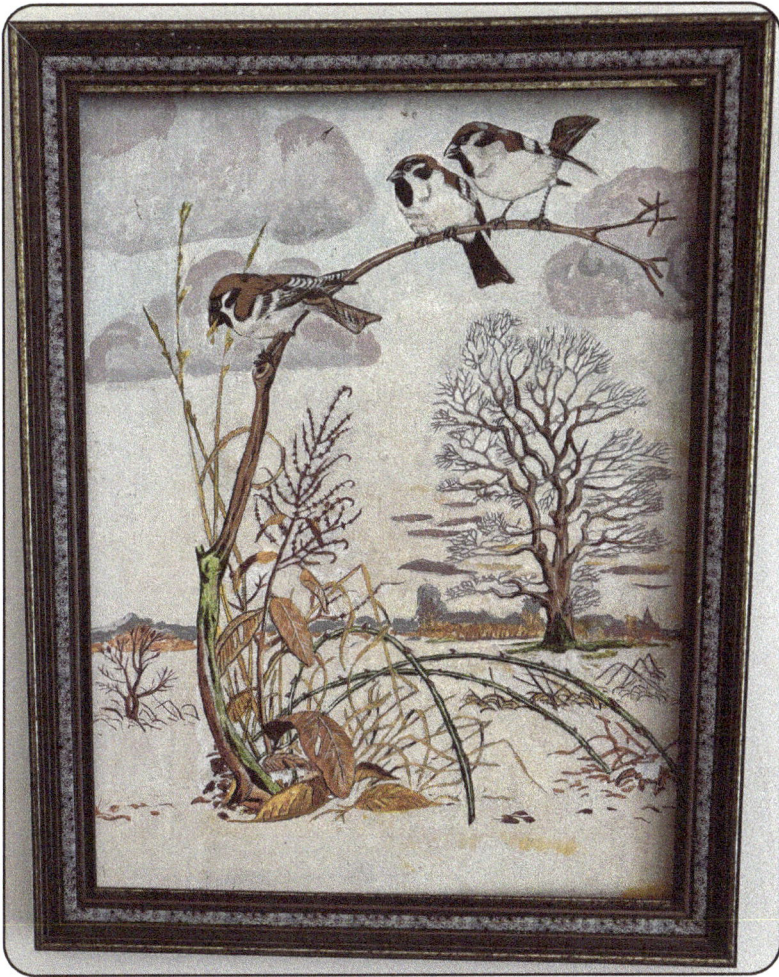

One of Nerida's first paintings at age 13 years old.

I spent only about a year in Sydney working as a cocktail barmaid. Back then, you did not have to prove your age, and I always looked very mature, so telling the boss that I was 18 was very believable. I also worked as a salesgirl in the Rocks in Sydney: the arts centre for hand-made artefacts. I had a little room in a huge old mansion in Double Bay with 10 other young people. Afterwards, I went on to rent a little flat on my own in the eastern suburbs of Sydney with my new dog, Kimba, whom I had rescued from terrible abuse. We loved each other, and he was the best company.

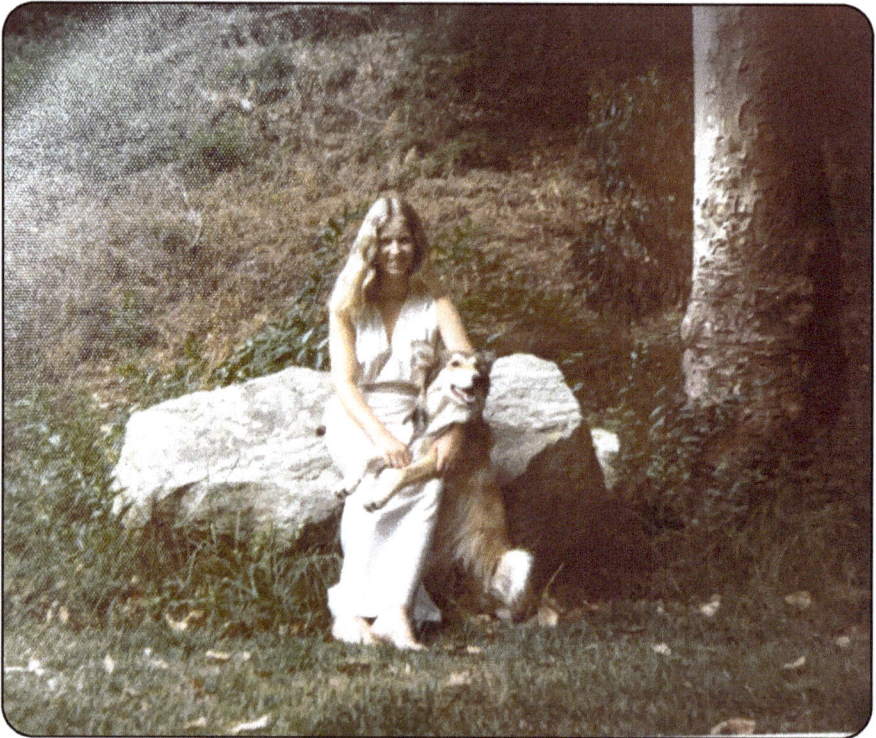

At 16, I moved to Wagga Wagga. Why? Because of a boy, of course. We wanted to get out of the city and live a more country life together.

At this point in my life, I was doing a lot of yoga, and I also discovered that I had a natural talent for massage. I would

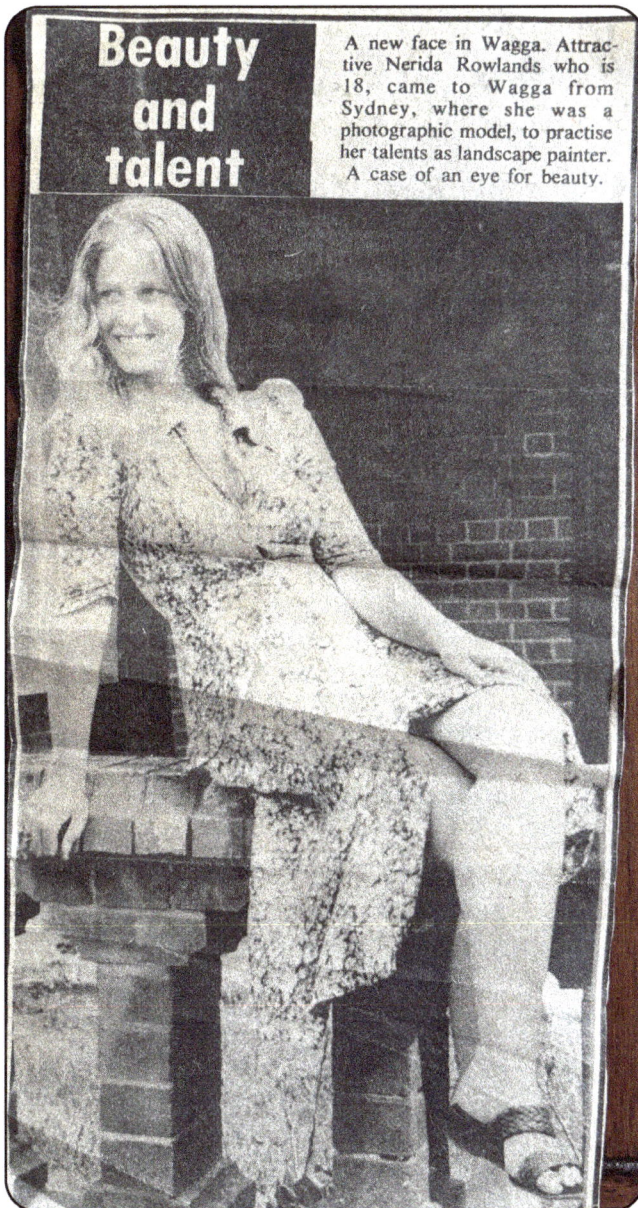

Beauty and talent

A new face in Wagga. Attractive Nerida Rowlands who is 18, came to Wagga from Sydney, where she was a photographic model, to practise her talents as landscape painter. A case of an eye for beauty.

practise deep tissue massage on whomever was around at the time and needed help. I soon began to realise that I loved helping people. I applied for a job with a chiropractor doing massage for his patients in readiness for chiropractic adjustments. There were three applicants, and we all had to give the chiropractor who was hiring a massage. The other two applicants were qualified, yet I got the job despite having no qualifications.

I remember my first four-day week, massaging 25 patients a day. For the first several days, I would come home at night and fall asleep in the armchair for two hours straight as soon as I sat down. I was exhausted!

After a short time, I noticed that whenever I was massaging, my hands would become so hot. Patients often asked if I had heated the massage oil. Whenever I stopped work, my hands would go cold again. I wondered, was this a special energy or was it just heat? I got a thermometer out one day and held it in between my hands when I was working, but the temperature was exactly the same as when my hands were cold. Strange…

I deduced this had to be a special energy, perhaps a healing energy. I then instinctively imagined that energy coming in through the top of my head and passing through my arms to my hands. If I could increase that energy, I thought, perhaps I won't be so tired by the end of the day by doing this. Much to my amazement, it worked, and I stopped being so worn out at the end of each day. To this day, 40+ years later, my reception staff say things to me like, "How do you have the stamina to give the same amount to each patient, at the end of a long day, as you do at the start?"

This first job in the health industry started me on my journey! It is a journey I am writing about now, four decades later.

After a year working with the chiropractor, I had begun adjusting spines, firstly on the chiropractor himself, and then the spines of friends – there weren't many practitioners around in a country town. I soon found out that I had a natural talent for this too. I recall him coaching me that very first time I did an adjustment.

Once I did that first neck adjustment, it was like it all came flooding back from somewhere. So strange, really. I felt completely comfortable doing manipulation of the spine and I could also envision the person's spine and see the touch, through my fingers, relaying the information back to my mind, exactly how their spine was misaligned. It was almost like X-ray vision; it is magical how easy this is for me to envision.

I have only ever needed X-rays for severe falls or car and motorbike accidents for my patients where there was a real risk of fractures. Otherwise, palpation on my patients (the placing of hands to feel and assess what is misaligned in the joints or spine) is and always has been my most accurate way of assessing what was needed to reduce their pain and gently realign the individual vertebrae.

I then moved onto another job in the health industry. I began working for an acupuncturist. He had five clinics all around NSW. I would work with him doing massage and adjustments on his patients, and then he would put in the acupuncture needles. I would go away every second week to the other four clinics around NSW and work every week in the Wagga clinic. Soon, his patients were just waiting for me to work on them, and he became busy only every second week. He became jealous and resentful of this, so I decided to find work elsewhere.

It was at that time I was invited to a Down to Earth Confest, a huge festival covering acres of farmland held on a country property somewhere in Victoria or NSW. Thousands attended and I ended up in the healing village treating about 40 people a day for three days straight during one of those festivals. Here, I got my internship, you might say, and gained enormous confidence in how much I could help people with both remedial massage and chiropractic adjustments.

It was then I met the politician Don Chip, who was the driving force behind these Confests. He was a big proponent of biodynamic farming and all things natural. He had a friend who offered his home in Sherbrooke Road in the Dandenong Ranges, Victoria, to the Down To Earth movement, for use in delivering workshops, and I was invited to help. I taught therapeutic massage workshops with others, along with organic vegetarian cooking classes. I loved this time of exploring the whole natural lifestyle approach.

So from Wagga Wagga, I packed up my life and hitchhiked to Victoria, to Ferny Creek Dandenong Ranges. I recall I was all of 17 by now, being picked up on the way by a very kind Mac truck driver who dropped me off in Sherbrooke Forest Road residence at the doorstep of my destination. It was late one night, and I recall being in this huge semi-trailer truck navigating these windy roads to my destination. The fog, the tree fern-covered roads, the enormous mountain ash gum trees: it was just magical. Back then, hitchhiking did not hold the dangers of today. The driver appreciated the company on the long drive as it helped him stay awake.

I remember awakening the next day, in my newfound bed in Sherbrooke forest, to the sound of bagpipes at the crack of dawn! "What… How?" I thought. I climbed out of bed in my lacy, white, vintage nightgown and barefoot, tiptoed out of the house to follow this hauntingly beautiful sound. Where on earth was this sound of bagpipes coming from in the middle of an Australian bush forest? I soon discovered I was close to the Baron of Beef, as it was known back then, which was just like a castle with about 125 rooms and blue stone with parapets. Here I found a man in full Scottish regalia, standing there playing his bagpipes in the early morning mist of the mountains. It felt like I was in fairyland.

It was then, as I looked around at the huge mountain ash gums, mixed with English oaks and many tall tree ferns – such magnificent greenery – I thought to myself, I would love to own a place up here one day. It was truly beautiful.

After six months living and working from this wonderful house in Sherbrooke Road, Don Chip's friend needed his house back. We moved the Down To Earth offices to Fitzroy, in the city of Melbourne, to a newly renovated building called the Universal Workshop – a big project which had 80 shops inside and a performance stage for local and international artists to showcase their music. Here, I started up my first small practice, doing massage and adjustments and giving some nutritional advice in the back room behind the Down To Earth office.

One time, a man was carried into my room. He had spent many hours creating paintings that adorned the dark blue walls covered with planets, universes and stars: both the inside and outside of this magnificent three-story old brick building. He had done his back in so badly that he could no longer even walk, which was no doubt from all the hours and hours of standing on ladders to paint his amazing artworks. After my treatment, he got up and walked out without any pain. We became close friends and after some weeks, months, and years, he went on to become the father of our two beautiful daughters, both of whom have ended up artists in their own right – as well as wonderful mothers of my five gorgeous grandchildren!

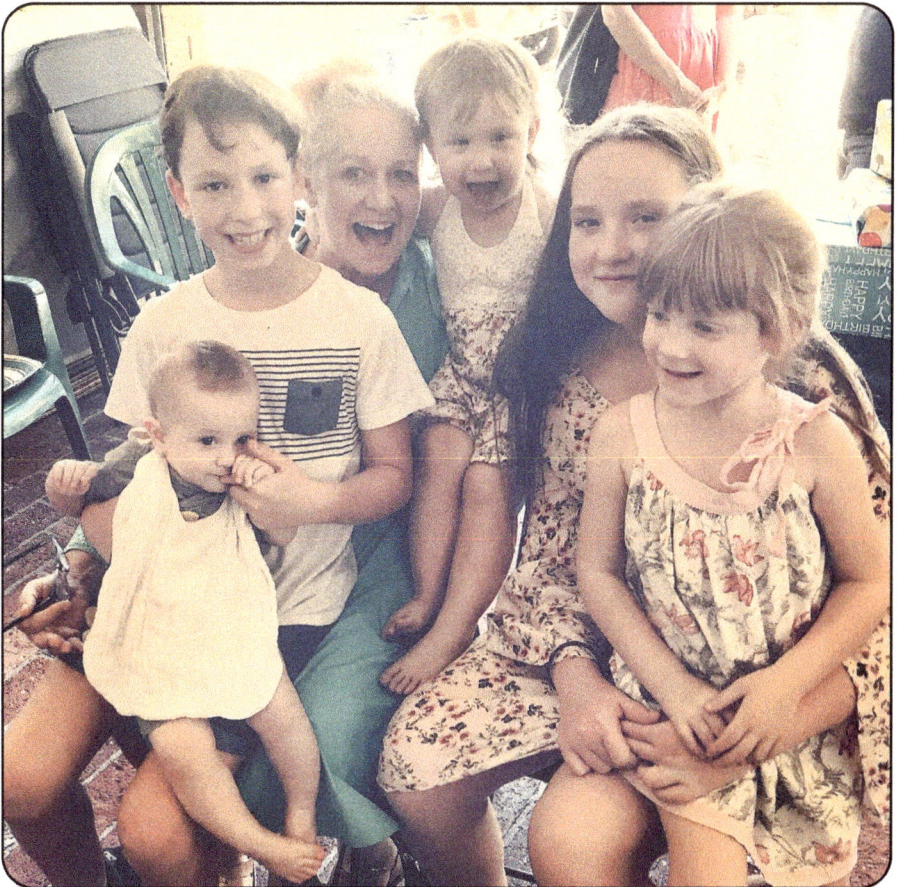

All this time, I was still suffering the acne and continued to suffer with doctors still saying, "She will grow out of it." But here I was, now 18 years old, and I had still not "grown out" of my acne. I had even tried the contraceptive pill, but it just made me feel nauseated, and my acne got even worse. It was during this time that I experienced the second significant awakening on my healing journey.

My stubborn acne motivated me to do my own research. So, I stopped eating red meat, stopped all dairy products (except butter), and I stopped wheat totally. Within weeks, there was a big difference in my skin. Six months later, my face had cleared up completely and I realised there was a lot to be said for the nutritional influence of what one ate and one's health. Hence the saying, "You are what you eat!"

After about 18 months working for the Down to Earth group, both in the hills and their Fitzroy offices, I ended up living in an old farmhouse in Gembrook, which was about 70 kilometres from Melbourne city centre. I moved my practice there while having my first baby. At this time, I was also working for a very progressive and alternative medical doctor in Collins Street in the Melbourne CBD. He needed someone to massage and adjust his patients for him while he practised alternative medicine using herbs and homeopathic remedies. He only prescribed medical drugs as a last resort for his patients. These GPs are known today as integrative medical doctors.

During this time, I also came upon a spiritual movement, a practical philosophy. This organisation fulfilled a search I felt I had been on since leaving home at such a young age, a search for a happier and more stable version of myself. It didn't seem right to be so happy one minute and so miserable the next. I was searching for greater stability and something more from life than mere survival…

One of the first things that I did was a sauna detox, the purpose being that if your body is cleared of the majority of chemicals you have ingested over the years, toxins, drugs – both medical or recreational drugs – and even alcohol, once these are cleared from the body, your perceptions and memory become sharper and clearer, all the better to assist any future counselling, and most definitely making the counselling much more effective. Let's face it: trying to counsel a person stoned, drunk, or high on mind-numbing psychiatric drugs just doesn't work!

Alcohol, recreational drugs, and even painkillers can inhibit our natural senses to a greater or lesser degree. Talk to any counsellor out there; counselling requires the ability to recall, remember and, at times, relive your past and its traumas, so as to clear them of the power they may still elicit over you at times. How can you clear past traumas if you can't recall your past? You can't achieve a greater awareness of self and life if you are clouded by mind-altering medications, drugs, or alcohol.

I noticed a big change after this sauna detox program. My emotional stability improved a lot, and my IQ went up 10 points. Not only did I feel extremely clean within my body, I had a renewed sense of wellbeing, almost like a cellular vitality. I loved this process and, as a result, decided that I wanted more knowledge and skills to help myself and others in their lives.

Over these early years, I had avoided my family all together. They just caused me emotional pain and feelings of invalidation, inadequacy, as well as triggering memories that I did not want to recall. However, this spiritual movement encouraged me to get back in touch with my mother and father. The counsellor coached me on how to speak with love and kindness and how to be more respectful, using warmth and common topics when speaking to them and to keep our conversations positive and constructive. This worked well, and I began to re-establish a relationship with them both, in their separate lives, after their divorce. I am very happy to say that I have now had long and warm relationships with them both.

During this process, I came to realise my own accountability in the family breakdown, and I educated myself about taking responsibility for my own emotions, actions, and behaviour in life. I have discovered that this is essential on the road to being truly happy.

I noticed that, as a result of this counselling, I went onto clear away a lot of the negative emotions and attitudes I had developed as a very young teenager. I became more able to help others, and my natural medicine clinic began to grow and grow. My energy was better, and I was able to work long hours with no adverse emotional effects. It was fantastic.

This spiritual movement also encouraged me at that time to get qualifications for my skills in nutrition and obtain certificates for my massage and manipulation chiropractic skills, since I was practising and consulting with patients, though not having studied for any formal qualifications. By that point, I was now pregnant with baby girl number two and still living in Gembrook.

At this stage, I was also in the midst of a course regarding the topic of how to study, which was an important part of this spiritual movement. This gave me study skills and opened my life to books. I became an avid reader for the first time in my life, my literacy improved yet again, and this also gave me the confidence to do a double degree.

I found a college in Ringwood, the Laws College of Naturopathy and Chiropractic, only 45 minutes from the farm I was living on and running my practice from. I went to see the principal of the college for an interview. Because I had left school early and had no high school certificate, which was a prerequisite to entry, I wanted to plead my case in person. I took along several of my patient files to demonstrate my experience in having treated patients for several years by that point. I implored the principal of the college to allow me to gain the qualifications so that I could conform to the laws of the land.

I explained to her that I was doing a professional study course and felt that I could cope with the two four-year degrees: one in Naturopathy and one in chiropractic. She agreed, much to my relief. I then went a step further and pushed my luck by convincing her into letting me do these double degrees in two years (not four) by paying double fees and attending double lectures and sitting double the exams. She agreed on the proviso that I would come to her and slow down if I felt I was not coping or if my grades were poor. I agreed. I then turned in 28 essays per year and did 32 exams per year. Or was it the other way around? Either way, it was a lot of work!

In that first year, I recall the class began with 60 students in attendance, but with only 12 students left by end of the fourth year: a huge dropout rate. But I had my study skills and excelled.

To this day, I look back and still wonder how I did all this with a five-month-old baby girl, a four-year-old daughter, running my practice four days a week, all whilst being the only breadwinner of this little family. Needless to say, it was tough, but I did it. I was the first student to ever achieve this, though, of course, I had no social life at all during those years.

I obtained my double degrees within those two years. I also received a certificate of homeopathy and a diploma of Iridology, plus I am recognised as a qualified remedial massage therapist, which was included within the Naturopathy degree. Not only did I achieve both my degrees, but I also stepped in and taught biochemistry to the first-year students when the college suddenly lost a lecturer.

I can't recall if it was a term or longer, but I stepped in to help until the department found a replacement. Teaching other students was also extremely helpful because you definitely had to know the theory of biochemistry to teach it, and since it was my least favourite subject, it gave me a good excuse to apply my skills to this challenge.

What was great about all this was that it was happening while I continued to treat my patients. I was able to put into practice each week everything I was learning, and I could apply it to my patients while it was still fresh in my mind, meaning a good balance of theory and practical application right through those two years!

Every day I still use this depth of knowledge to investigate the cause of a patient's symptoms rather than just treating the symptom itself.

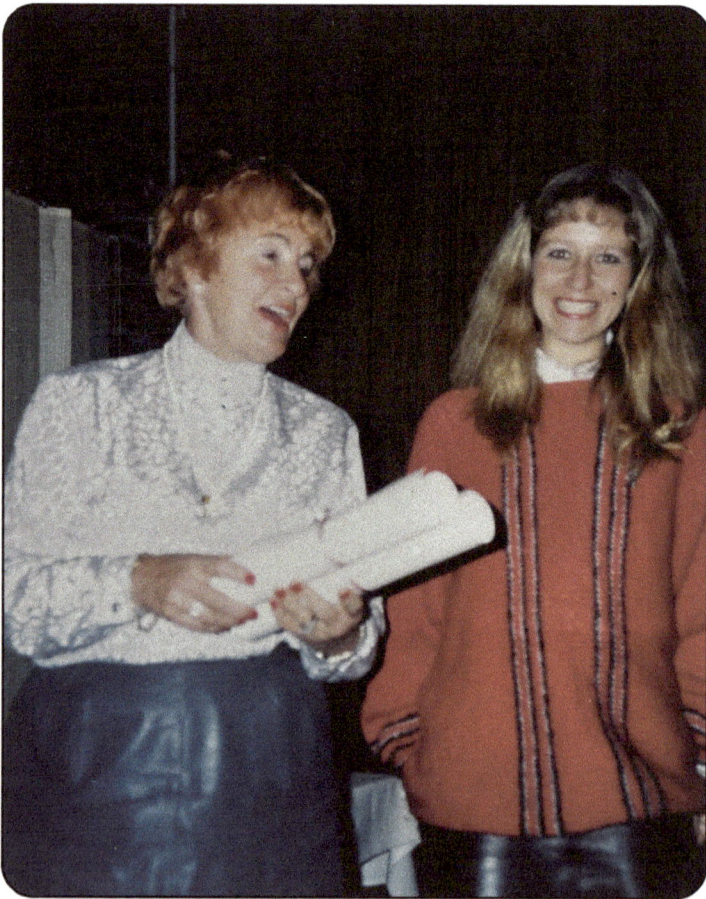

Nerida receiving her 3rd year certificates.

Laws College For Naturopathy

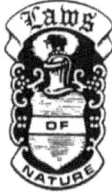

does hereby certify that

Nerida B. James

having completed the prescribed curriculum and passed the Final Examinations in

Homoeopathic Medicine

is granted this Certificate

Duration of this course is 12 months.

20·12·1987.

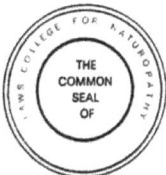

P. J. Laws N.D. IR.D MOH. D

Principal &C. IR. I4

Registrar

Certificate No. **77·**

THE COMMON SEAL OF

Laws College for Naturopathy

Whereas **Nerida B. James**

has completed the practical and theory studies prescribed by this college and has passed the requisite examinations to determine qualification in the

Department of Naturopathic Medicine

Now Therefore she has been conferred by this college with the diploma of

Naturopathy (N.D.)

and declared a Graduate of the LAWS COLLEGE

"THREE YEAR COURSE"
Given under the Seal of the College
this 14 day of June A.D. 1987

Certificate No. 86

Principal
Registrar

Laws College Naturopathy & Chiropractic

Whereas **Nerida B. James**

has completed the practical and theory studies prescribed by this College and has passed the requisite examinations to determine qualification in the

Department of Naturopathic Medicine

Now Therefore she has been conferred by this College with the degree of

Bachelor of Naturopathy (N.D.)

and declared a Graduate of the LAWS COLLEGE

"FOUR YEAR COURSE"

Given under the Seal of the College
this 20 day of Dec. A.D. 1987.

Certificate No. 104.

Principal
Registrar

Laws College For Naturopathy

Whereas **Nerida B. James**

has completed the THREE YEARS practical and theory studies prescribed by this College and has passed the requisite examinations to determine qualification in the

Department of Iridology

Now Therefore **she** has been conferred by this College with the Diploma of

Iridology (Dip. Irid.)

and declared a Graduate of the LAWS COLLEGE

Given under the Seal of the College
this **14** day of **JUNE** A.D. **1987**

Principal

Registrar

Certificate No. **86**

Laws College

Naturopathy & Chiropractic

Whereas **Nerida B. James**

has completed the practical and theory studies prescribed by this College and has passed the requisite examinations to determine qualification in the

Department of Chiropractic

Now Therefore **she** has been conferred by this College with the degree of

Bachelor of Chiropractic (D.C.)

and declared a Graduate of the LAWS COLLEGE
"FOUR YEAR COURSE"

Given under the Seal of the College
this **20** day of **Dec.** A.D. **1987**

Principal

Registrar

Certificate No. **105.**

1999
Australian
Achiever
A W A R D S
For Melbourne's
Health Services

Highly Commended

For excellence in customer relations
Awarded to

NERIDA JAMES NATURAL HEALING CENTRE

Administrating Director   Administrating Director

3AK
AM 1303
The Australian Achiever Network

Laws College of Naturopathy

HIPPOCRATIC OATH

(Modified)

To consider dear to me as my parents him who taught me this art of NATUROPATHY, to live in common with him and if necessary to share my goods with him, to look upon his children as my own brothers, to teach them this art if they so desire without fee or written promise, to impart to my sons and the sons of the master who taught me and the disciples who have enrolled themselves and have agreed to the rules of the profession, but to these alone, the precepts and the instruction. I will prescribe regimen for the good of my patients according to my ability and my judgement and never do harm to anyone. To please no one will I prescribe drugs or perform surgical operations nor give advice which may cause his death. Nor will I give a woman medication to procure abortion. But I will preserve the purity of my life and my art. I will not cut for stone, even for patients in whom the disease is manifest; I will leave this operation to be performed by practitioners (specialists in this art). To co-operate and if necessary refer patients to medical practitioners, and centres for tests. Every patient that enters my clinic and every house where I come only for the good of my patients, keeping myself far from all intentional ill-doing and all seduction, and especially from the pleasures of love with women or with men. All that may come to my knowledge in the exercise of my profession or outside of my profession or in daily commerce with men, which ought not to be spread abroad, I will keep secret and will never reveal. If I keep this oath faithfully, may I enjoy my life and practice my art, respected by all men and in all times; but if I swerve from it or violate it, may the reverse be my lot.

Hippocrates of Cos — Greece (island)
late 5th century — the famous Greek physician who is generally regarded as the "father of medicine".

Signature of final year student

Date 15 - 12 - 87   Date 15 - 12 - 87

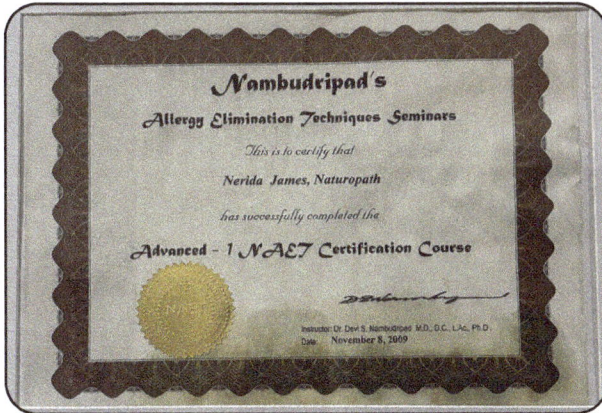

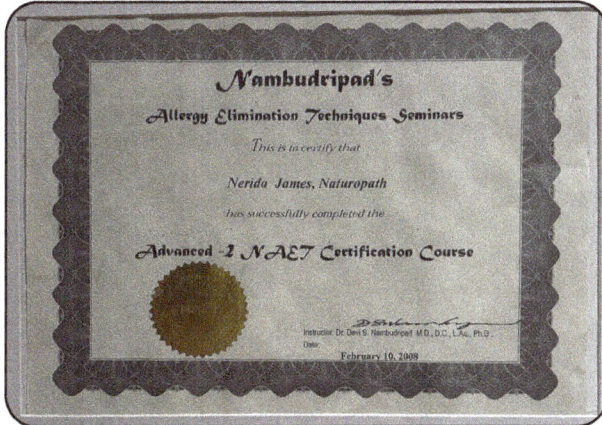

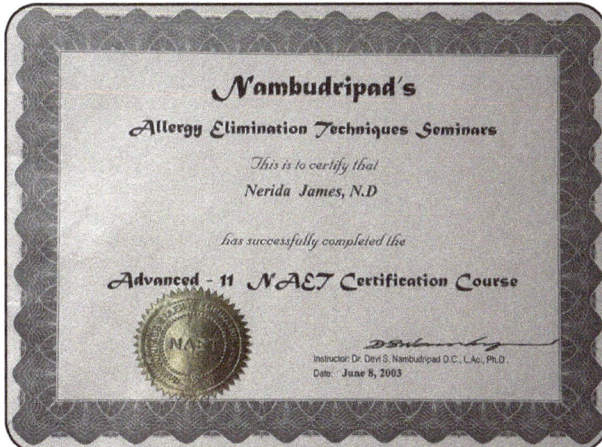

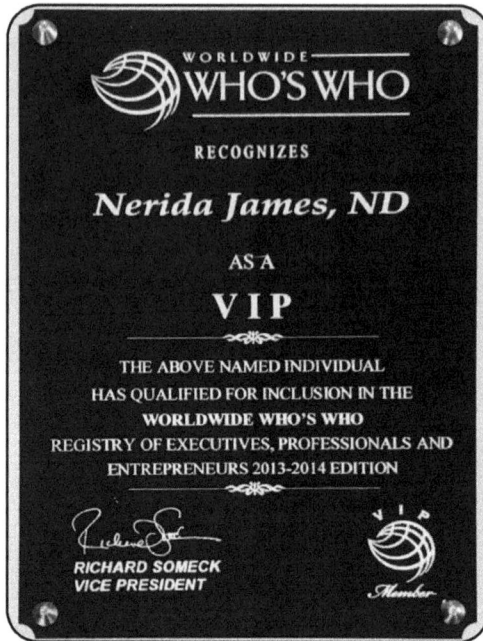

WORLDWIDE
WHO'S WHO

RECOGNIZES

Nerida James, ND

AS A

VIP

THE ABOVE NAMED INDIVIDUAL
HAS QUALIFIED FOR INCLUSION IN THE
WORLDWIDE WHO'S WHO
REGISTRY OF EXECUTIVES, PROFESSIONALS AND
ENTREPRENEURS 2013-2014 EDITION

**RICHARD SOMECK
VICE PRESIDENT**

VIP
Member

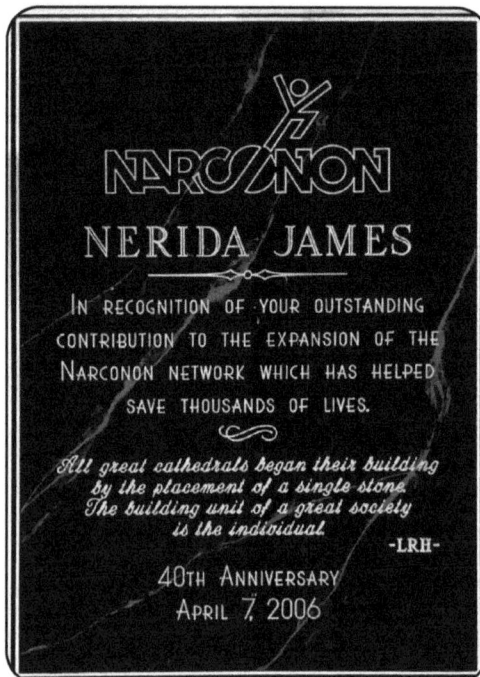

NARCONON

NERIDA JAMES

IN RECOGNITION OF YOUR OUTSTANDING
CONTRIBUTION TO THE EXPANSION OF THE
NARCONON NETWORK WHICH HAS HELPED
SAVE THOUSANDS OF LIVES.

*All great cathedrals began their building
by the placement of a single stone.
The building unit of a great society
is the individual.*

-LRH-

40TH ANNIVERSARY
APRIL 7, 2006

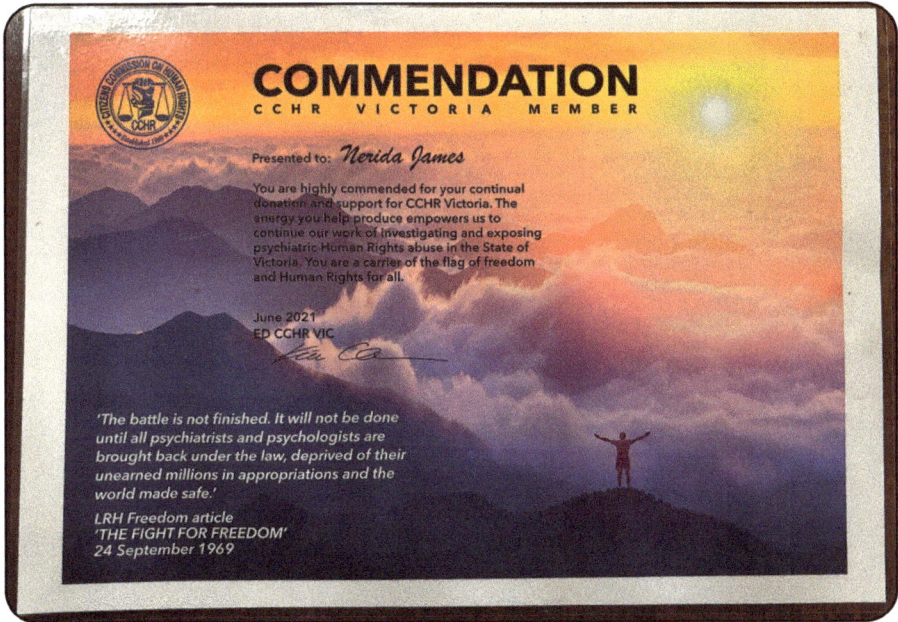

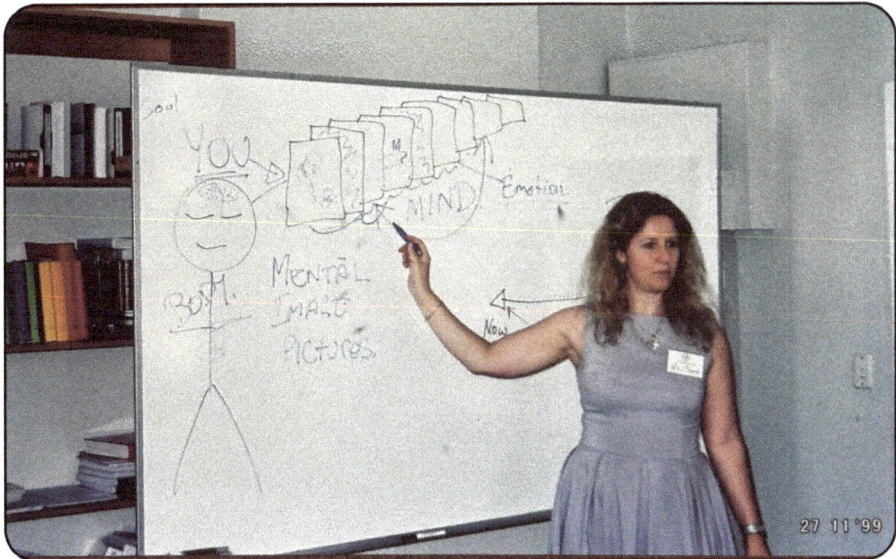

Nerida giving a lecture on drugs and their effects on the mind at her Get Off Drugs Naturally offices.

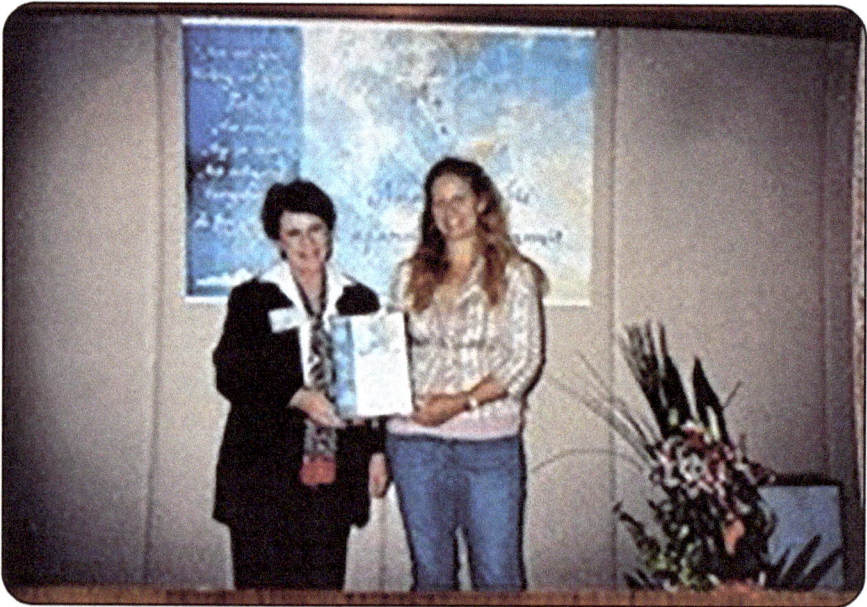

Nerida receiving an award for her humanitarian work in drug and alcohol rehabilitation.

In the year 2000 I went onto open and run, as a director, a drug and alcohol rehabilitation facility and this was my charity work for 20 years to come. This was a get off drugs naturally program which achieved wonderful success. But that is a story all of its own!

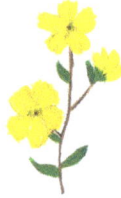

1

Take Your Power Back for Lasting Wellness

If you are unwell and tired, feel flat and overwhelmed with life, then, to address this, there has to be a change in your own mindset.

For how was it that you got into this situation, this health picture in the first place?

Is it your doctor's fault? No...

Is it your parents' fault? Maybe...

Is it your genes' fault, the parts of your body you inherited? Maybe...

Is it your education's fault? Maybe...

Is it your own fault? Yes...

The answer must be yes if you are ever going to get out of the situation you find yourself in. The willingness to look, search, learn, and find out the WHY behind the reason you are not in good health all starts with you. You are the master of your own destiny not just in your job, your choice of clothing, but most definitely in your own good health. I realised at a young age that in order to be happy, I must also be healthy.

Which, I was not, as I mentioned in my story above. The desire, that strong desire to take control of my health was the driving force in how I handled my own acne at the age of 18. And that desire, that driving force, has been with me in all my years. At times, of course we fall over, as I have, and throw ourselves on the bed and cry, sometimes feeling like giving up. It's just all too hard.

But you must hone in and harness the survival instinct to pick yourself up and keep trying, keep going, and keep looking, and one day you WILL find a way to make life easier and regain your health and personal power to be the best YOU you can be.

I believe educating yourself is a powerful way to start. If you have the know-how of something, then you cannot be the adverse effect of that something as a wise man once said! I know this to be true, as when you fully learn how to drive a car, you don't cause accidents, and when you take your car in for a regular service, then it doesn't break down.

Your body is very much the same way. If you learn how to care for it, how to give it a regular service, then guess what? It does NOT break down, and its power is just as good 20 years, 30 years, or 40 years later – and even beyond that. The one thing a body has over your car, however, is it can regenerate itself and renew itself, and it does so all the time. How do you think a cut on your finger heals? How does that broken bone heal? How does your body grow?

Learning to trust your own immune system, your own innate healing power of your body is not something we are taught anywhere, at any time in our life. We just get told what to do by our parents, by our schoolteachers, by social media, and by the internet.

Never are we given a very clear education about our body or its inner workings, nor our relationship as spiritual beings with our body or what it's really about. So we just go along, hoping for the best, and when we are broken down and suffering or injured and ill, we turn up and say, "Hey doc, fix me."

But guess what? You have a lot to do with whether or not you will get well. There may be times when we are faced with a dramatic disaster, and this makes us wake up and take stock of our life and what we were doing. Unfortunately, too many of us just blindly go along with life, just hoping for the best, hoping we won't get cancer, hoping we won't get sick like the next-door neighbour did.

I am here to tell you – you can be the one who says, "No, this is not happening to me. I am going to be responsible and take charge of my own body. I am going to make sure it is going to last me the next 80 or 90 years."

You can have great energy when you are 70, 80, and even 90. Your decisions and your attitude to yourself and your body make the difference. Of course, your determination to change your 'modus operandi' is also a vital ingredient to success.

By changing your way of living – and by this, I mean identifying and altering whatever you have been doing that has led you to this point of ill health – is a vital step in regaining your health. Logic dictates if you don't change something, you are going to continue on that path which leads you to sickness or destruction. Running scared of your body and just leaving it up to the experts is a surefire way to land yourself in more hot water. If your body is giving you a warning sign and you don't take heed, then you are headed in the wrong direction.

I'll give some examples of this throughout this book. By teaching even some basics, I find, as the years go by, my patients often know what to do if a symptom turns up, and they even end up helping their friends and family with basic knowledge of good health habits and practices.

I've said to both my daughters at times when I have overheard them talking to a friend, "You sound just like a Naturopath with that advice you just gave." I guess that years of living with the knowledge and applying it to themselves and their lives means they can now take control of their own health and inspire others to do the same.

And that is my wish for you: to take control of your health and wellbeing and come out the winner, not only helping yourself, but those around you. I believe all knowledge should be freely given and no practitioner or doctor should hide their successful actions, ever. Let's face it though: there are so many sick people in this world, no health professional will ever be out of work.

A final word on this subject: LISTEN TO YOUR INTUITION.

If something doesn't feel right for you, then don't do it — and not because you think it's too hard, though, that should never be a reason — but because that voice we all have inside us is telling you something is not right. So always do yourself a favour, and listen to that voice!

And with that, enjoy these chapters, follow the advice and take what you feel is right from them to help both yourself and those around you.

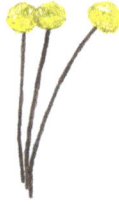

2

My Philosophy for Lasting Wellness

After 45 years in practice, I wish to leave a legacy of the work, knowledge, and experience I have gained to share with as many people as possible. Along with my additional training in the Bowen technique, Alexander posture correction, drug withdrawal training, Nambudripad's Allergy Elimination Technique (NAET) and the Lester Cox technique of ligament manipulation, I wish to impart my understanding of the human body and our underlying causes of disease, whether they be emotional, spiritual, or most importantly, physical in nature.

I believe this knowledge can open the door to help manage and resolve our suffering in the world today. Disease, or dis-ease as we refer to it in Naturopathy, is exactly that: a feeling of being ill at ease with our body and a discomfort which can range from mild to severe. We can call it pain.

In Naturopathy, there are five laws of nature that if violated, can lead to disease states of varying degrees. I've laid them out here for you:

1. **Drink enough pure water** – How many of us don't drink enough water? And, when we do, how pure is that water? Is it packed with chemicals put into it to kill bacteria? Chemicals to strengthen our teeth – as apparently our body does not know how to have strong teeth? Mountain spring water untouched by industry provides us with oxygen, hydrogen, and minerals, so drinking purified unadulterated water is vital for good health.

   See RESOURCE 1: Body Water Functions

2. **Eat fresh, natural food** – This means live, vital, pure food, with no processing or additives, no preservatives, no artificial colours, no artificial flavours, and food storage of minimum time frames. Ideally, eat organic food where the soil quality is usually much better. **Remember, pesticides kill the good bacteria in your gut.**

   See RESOURCE 2: My Healthy Diet Sheet

3. **Get enough sleep** – How many of us do not get enough sleep since the invention of the electric light? Our days now go until 11pm at night before we can sit down for

some *me* time. Bed can be midnight or 1am, then we are up at 5am or 6am to get ourselves and our family off to work, school, or the gym. The human body is meant to get seven to eight hours of sleep a night, and young children, who are growing at a rapid rate, need nine to twelve hours in bed to get enough sleep. This is important for memory, learning, and emotional stability.

See RESOURCE 3: My Sleep Hygiene Resource Sheet

4. **Exercise regularly** – With the invention of the automobile, trains, buses, and planes, many of us work hard and long hours and suffer from little to no exercise. We lie in our beds, we sit in our cars, we sit at our desks, and we sit on our couches. This lack of movement was never meant for the human body. It does very well with physical work, exercise, and stretching. I recommend a minimum of an hour three times a week but even more than this is better.

5. **Rest and Relaxation** – This includes social interaction with family, friends, and groups we are part of. We are very social beings and flourish when we are together. This can even include counselling or any form of activity to calm and bring peace to oneself. It could also be some form of creative expression such as music, art, painting, walks

along the beach, singing to oneself, doing a jigsaw puzzle, anything.

However, many of us don't do one or more of these five laws of nature. It is not uncommon for me to see a patient who lives on takeaways or readymade microwave meals containing denatured processed foods, who drinks little to no water but lots of coffee and alcohol, who doesn't get enough sleep due to long days and early mornings, who does not exercise, and who has little time to themselves for rest and relaxation.

They then wonder why they are always tired with headaches, or they feel anxious and sometimes depressed and unfulfilled in life. I see them overwhelmed, with life running them, instead of them running their own life and life choices. It sounds simplistic, but I can often trace their health issues back by beginning with the neglect of themselves in one or more of the five laws of nature. Perhaps it's the desire for financial gain or the caring of everyone else instead of themselves? However, neglecting a balance and not looking after oneself as well as others often ends in tears!

There is now a *new* health problem being bandied around known as burnout syndrome. Is it any wonder, with not enough sleep, not enough water, no exercise, and being so stressed that people can barely think or function well? These five laws of nature are fundamental when approaching a patient, whether it be with cancer, an autoimmune disease, or just a general malaise that cannot be diagnosed by a blood test, X-rays, ultrasound, or MRI scans.

This brings me to the title of this book, *Which Doctor?* There is a place for all doctors in our world. These days, we can also enjoy the marvellous surgical advances for those needing joint replacements, those who have experienced severe accidents, and others who need life-saving procedures. All of these practices are important and sometimes vital for the survival of a patient. However, I would say there are too many practitioners of all kinds with *extremist attitudes* that say *their* modality is the only way for all patients in all walks of life.

My philosophy is there is a place for us all when it comes to health and wellbeing. In fact, the merging of allopathic medicine (drugs and surgery) with natural medicine (naturopathy, homeopathy, osteopathy, chiropractic, and acupuncture to name a few) is the way of the future.

After 45 years in practice, the one-recipe-fits-all approach or any cookie-cutter treatment plan is a very blinkered and simplistic view, which leaves many ill patients wondering, "Who do I go to next to get help? The GP says there is nothing wrong; the specialist has discharged me from their care saying there is nothing wrong, but I still have pain, and I am still suffering the same symptoms."

This brings me to why wrote this book, **Which Doctor?**

I had a classic case of this recently when a dentist came in as an emergency patient. She had woken up in the middle of the night around 3.30am, not feeling too well. She took herself to the bathroom and had an episode where she could hardly breathe, felt faint with chest pain on her left side, and pain down her arm. She almost passed out. Her words to me were "I thought I was going to die." She managed to get herself back to her bed where she then asked her husband to call an ambulance. The emergency services spoke to her on the phone for an hour while the ambulance was meant to be arriving.

In the meantime, her husband got her some of the natural medicine she had been prescribed by myself nine months earlier. She took a high-dose probiotic for soothing the gut and digestive medicine. She started to feel better. As the ambulance had still not arrived, she told them not to come as she wanted to sleep. They then advised her to see her GP the next morning.

She went to work, saw a few patients, and then went to her GP. He checked her blood pressure and her heart and then recommended she go to a hospital to get blood tests and a scan. She still had the pain in her chest and the top of her left arm, but it was not as debilitating as the previous night. The GP gave her a report, which she showed me, where it stated there was no evidence of a heart attack, but he felt that her symptoms should be investigated further.

It turns out that she had undergone a very similar event three months earlier and went to a specialist cardiologist back then, so she had already had the blood tests done for cardiac arrest, as well as an ECG, which all showed everything normal and that her heart was healthy. So, in her mind, she could not see the sense in repeating all these tests yet again just to be told there was nothing wrong.

She decided – and I quote – "Dr Nerida will know what is wrong with me. I'm seeing her first." I advised her to follow her GP's request as instructed because new blood tests would not lead her astray or do her any harm. After asking some more questions, I discovered she had eaten birthday cake with a lot of cream, sugar, and white wheat flour that night just before bed.

What had in fact happened was that she had experienced a severe allergic type of reaction, almost anaphylactic in severity, which in turn had severely spasmed her digestive tract and her upper back. Consequently, this had caused impingement of the nerves to her left arm and chest, due to the upper-back thoracic vertebrae being contracted when the muscle spasms occurred, leading to compression of the nerves descending from her spine to her arm and chest. We call this referred pain.

Knowing your anatomy and physiology well would logically suggest IF her heart is okay and her arteries are not compromised, the next thing to check would be nerve supply to the chest and arms – common sense really. For her treatment, I used a specialised technique called Nambudripad's Allergy Elimination Technique (NAET), which is a Chinese medicine-based acupressure treatment, for her wheat and dairy intolerance. Then I conducted some deep-tissue massage, realigned her upper back, tractioned her neck, and finally did some occipital release, which alleviates spasming around the base of the skull to promote better circulation to her brain.

I also discovered she was very underslept (which was a chronic problem for her) and as a dentist, she always had a lot of tension in her upper back and neck due to working over patients' mouths, bent over all day in the dental chair with her arms elevated. Her prescription was to stay off wheat and dairy and come back with her blood tests to follow up on her progress. Also, to get more sleep and do more exercise, especially stretching (I particularly love Pilates), to help the tension in the spine. She left the clinic that night, pain-free and with a big smile on her face, offering words of gratitude.

I have seen this type of scenario many, many times over in the last 40+ years, and in some cases, I have had patients fly from the other side of the country as a last resort because no one they had seen was able to assist with their condition or even accurately diagnose their cause. I sometimes call myself the last-resort doctor, and I welcome these patients as it is a challenge that I love. The wins are tremendous when you can turn around their lives and see the sparkle come back to their eyes over the course of just one session.

The other philosophy I have adapted is, if a case seems very complex, the practitioners in charge are missing something fundamental in that case.

An example of this was many years ago, when a patient presented at our clinic with a chronic asthma-type cough. She had been like this for eight or nine months and three of these months she had spent in hospital, undergoing many, many, blood tests, scans, X-rays, and MRIs. She had been given a plethora of drugs, much of which involved asthma medications and high doses of cortisone – none of which she responded to.

Her cough was so persistent and debilitating that it kept her awake most of the night. She was crying; she could barely speak to me without coughing about every two to three minutes. You can imagine how exhausted she was. She had been discharged by the hospital only to be told that her issue was psychosomatic: "You need to see a psychiatrist," along with a prescription for antidepressants, sleeping tablets, and a referral.

When she came to me, I listened to her, and I did some iridology, or iris diagnosis, which revealed severe bronchial and lung inflammation. It was then my job to find out why. I checked her spine for impingement of blood or nerve supply to her lungs/bronchioles, and while I found everything very tight from all the coughing, I found no severe impingement.

I then tested for allergies/intolerances with neurosensitivity testing, also known as muscle testing. I checked for food intolerances, then environmental sensitivities, viruses and/or bacterial infections. Nothing came up until I tested for fungal infection, specifically Aspergillus fumigatus, which is often found in air-conditioning units and potting mix. It turned out she worked in a nursery and was exposed to potting mix frequently. Now I had a cause!

Fungal infections do not show in blood tests, and this had not shown up in a sputum test either. I gave her a high dose of magnesium to calm down the broncho-spasming she was experiencing. I prescribed anti-fungal herbal medicines such as paud'arco, garlic, grapefruit seed extract, oregano oil, and thyme oil, along with herbs to boost her immune system, including olive leaf, astragalus, andrographis, goldenseal, blue flag, Japanese mushrooms, and vitamin C with polygonum.

We then applied the NAET technique for fungus sensitivity, especially the Aspergillus fumigatus with her lung meridian and bronchus. She was so sensitive to the fungal spores that it took eight sessions to get her body desensitised to the Aspergillus, all the while treating her fungal infestation in the lungs with herbs, homeopathics, and diet.

We changed her eating habits to help stop feeding the infection by taking her off concentrated sugars, all mucus-forming foods (largely wheat and dairy products), and I gave her herbs to calm her nervous system. Her body had become so hypersensitive due to the inflammation and lack of restorative sleep. All the while she was improving throughout her treatment which took three months of intensive therapy, but we did it: we finally got that cough to stop. As you can imagine, it had ruined her life. To see her day-to-day life restored back to some form of normality was the most rewarding thing for me as a practitioner.

Over the years, I have come to learn even the most severely ill patients can often be helped beyond my wildest dreams. So, these days, I just get the story of their illness, look for anomalies or information that doesn't seem to fit, check all their tests results, do my iris diagnosis, and just start with the basics. You would be surprised just how much and how fast the human body can bounce back from illness.

Sometimes being a good diagnostician is being like a detective using all your intelligence, experience, and know-how of the body as a whole: its anatomy and physiology. This also includes taking into account both mental stress and spiritual stress caused by a person in the patient's vicinity... an associate perhaps, that doesn't want to see them do well in life.

The importance here is really listening to the patient who is in front of you, like a clean slate being filled with their life's story: this cannot be overstated. Rapport is vital to earn the patient's trust so that they have faith in you when you give them a program. They leave with a sense of enthusiasm and hope about becoming well and healthy. I often say goodbye to a new patient after their visit with, "I look forward to getting you well and healthy!"

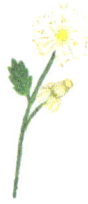

3

Iridology – Iris Diagnosis, A Dying Art

Iridology or iris diagnosis is a fundamental and important tool of the Naturopath. In my day, we did two years of training on this subject within our four-year degree. We used the textbook *Iridology-The Science and Practice of the Healing Arts* by Bernard Jensen. In the Naturopathic courses of today, it is either not offered or is an elective that is taught for one semester only, sometimes even less.

This is very sad for me, as without one of the fundamental diagnostic tools of a Naturopath being taught, a practitioner is relying solely on symptoms or relying on medical blood testing, which, if ordered by the Naturopath or alternative practitioner, is not covered by your healthcare here in Australia. Hence, the costs to the patient can be quite high, not to mention not always finding the cause of a patient's malady either. I do use functional pathology testing at times, along with blood tests, but I primarily rely on my iridology for diagnostic purposes along with taking down a thorough case history.

Here is an example; a patient comes into the clinic complaining of headaches. There could be 20 reasons this patient may have headaches. Do you just give a headache pill, or do you investigate the underlying CAUSE? Investigate always is my philosophy.

This is what Iridology can greatly assist with!

Headaches may be caused by liver toxicity, food allergies, spinal impingement of nerves, kidney underfunction or muscular tension or just plain stress and too many thoughts constantly going round and round, not allowing the person proper rest. Iridology used as a diagnostic tool can assist the Naturopathic practitioner to narrow down the reason why the patient is suffering.

This is for the Naturopathic practitioner that really cares and is willing to spend the time with their patients to fully understand the complete health picture. They are going to be a very successful practitioner. I have come to understand after many years of treating patients that accurate diagnosis means you are 80% there in terms of assisting or even completely resolving a patient's condition.

What is Iridology?

Iridology is an ancient technique of enlarging and studying the iris, the coloured part of the eye. It can guide the Naturopathic physician towards the underlying causative factor of a patient's symptoms.

By assessing both the colour and patterns of the fibres the iris is made up of, it gives a detailed picture to the Naturopathic physician about their patient's state of health. It does this by showing the reflex messaging back to the iris conditions of the body. However, it does *not* diagnose disease names! Meaning it won't, by modern medical categories, name out a disease, for example diabetes, in this case it may show the pancreas area in iridology is dark and under functioning or it may show that the area is inflamed and overactive. So now one can direct the patient for further testing to see is it hypoglycaemia or hyperglycaemia (diabetes) or is it type one or type two diabetes?

What it does show are things such as inflammation, under-activity of an area of the body, and the cellular vitality or weakness in certain body tissues or organs. This can reveal such things as leaky gut (medically known as dysbiosis) or the possibility of deficiencies of nutrients leading to the cause of a patient's symptoms. It can even show genetic inherited weaknesses, often verified by the patient's family history. I sometimes see a pancreas weakness, a sign showing pancreatic under-activity. If the sign in the iris shows a circular border all around the sign and it is a *thick* border, it often indicates an *inherited weakness* from a parent with diabetes. If it is a *thin* border, it could be an inherited weakness from a grandparent with diabetes.

A patient often looks amazed when I ask whether their mother or father has diabetes, and sure enough, it is confirmed with a positive "Yes!" Or I will ask, "Do you have a grandparent with diabetes?" and yes, it is confirmed by my patient that they do.

We can then approach this by strengthening that area of that patients' body, long before it becomes diseased. We call this *preventative medicine.*

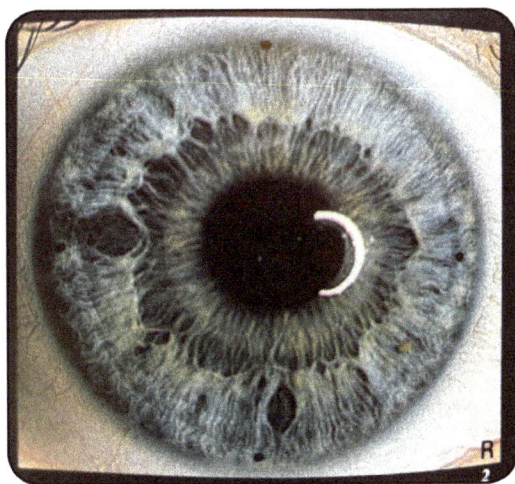

The almond-shaped sign at 6 o'clock...an underactive kidney.

Another example of what iridology can show would be the presence of nerve rings or cramp rings in the iris. These often indicate a patient's need for more magnesium, need for massage, stretching exercises, and possibly more relaxation or sleep. This sign, in the iris, is an indicator of nervous stress finding its way into the muscular system, brain, or even digestive system of the person.

After three or more months, we can then rephotograph their iris to show the patient's improvement due to all their hard work. Instead of three nerve rings, there may be one or none. Instead of severe inflammation, the iris looks a better colour and not as inflamed. It is also often confirmed by the patients themselves telling me their pain is greatly reduced. I saw this only the other day with a patient that has come back to the practice after many years, and we compared the now-to-the-then photos, and the difference was very discernible.

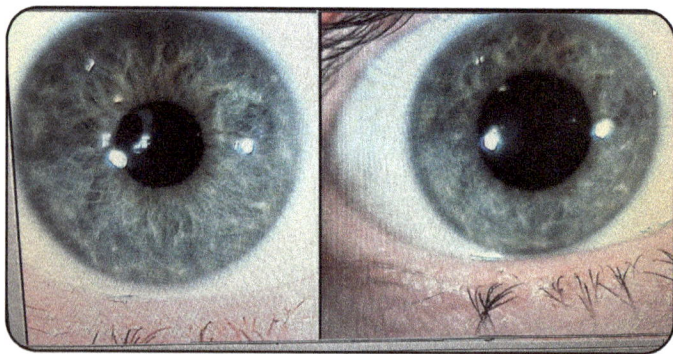

Here is an example on the left of the patient looking a lot better, the pupil being smaller and more even, indicating nervous exhaustion has gone.

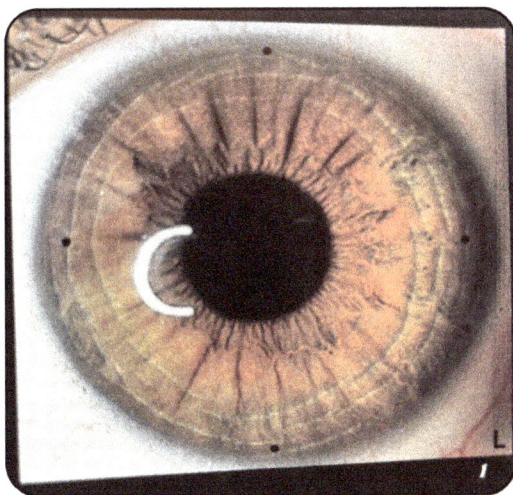

Here is an example of two-and-a-half nerve rings or cramp rings, the lines running around the iris.

Nature has provided us with an invaluable insight into the vital status of the health of our body by transmitting this information to the eye. To the practitioner, this can be extremely helpful in knowing how quickly a patient will respond to your recommended treatment protocol and most importantly, the underlying cause of their symptomology. As a side benefit, this is a very inexpensive, fast, and a non-invasive diagnostic technique.

The history of iridology is an interesting one that dates back to the 1870s. According to a German iridologist, the first documented reference can be credited to the physician Philippus Meyers who wrote the book *Chromatic Medica* published in Dresden, which describes parts of the iris representing parts of the body. A century later, yet another practitioner of medicine published a paper called *The Eye and it Signs.*

But considered the true originator of this science was Dr Ignatz Von Peczely (1826-1911). As a young Hungarian boy of 11 years old, he was trying to free an owl trapped in his garden and accidentally broke its leg. He soon noticed the appearance of a dark strip in the lower part of its eye. He then nursed the owl back to health. Later, he released the bird only to find it stayed in his garden for several years afterwards. He noticed, in the owl's eye, the appearance of a white crooked line which had developed exactly where the dark strip had been when he broke its leg. This phenomenon made a lasting impression on the young boy.

When he became older, Peczely became a homeopathic doctor (later a medical doctor) and while practising, he started to notice the differences and similarities in his patients' eyes. Fascinated by whether he would be able to discover anything significant, he began studying the eyes of his patients. He started observing and documenting the correlations between markings in the eyes and his patients' illnesses. These patterns in the iris of his patients' eyes led him to start using the eye as a diagnostic tool.

To identify different parts of the iris, Peczely described the different points as if looking at the face of a clock. As an example, he realised patients with kidney disease all had dark areas of the iris just inside the 6pm mark on a clock face. If it was liver disease, it would look dark approximately at 8pm on a clock face, but if it was hepatitis, it would appear white at 8pm.

He collected these records and began to develop the first in-depth eye chart showing his observations. His fame and success of using this unique art spread across his native land Budapest, where he was practising, and then later throughout Europe. Patients began to flock to him from all over the continent and it is said the birth of iridology was approximately in 1861.

Peczely's work was continued by at least 10 other practitioners over the following hundred years, many of whom were medical practitioners, osteopaths, chiropractors, and Naturopaths. They published papers and many books on iridology over the century, establishing the fundamental basics that come with iris diagnosis or iridology.

A very astute chiropractor and nutritionist named Dr Bernard Jenson picked up and studied the iridology work of many of these doctors and practitioners. As well as being mentored alongside some of these doctors, years later Dr Jenson wrote his own text called *Iridology: The Science and Practice in the Healing Arts*. This is the text I personally studied from and I have relied heavily on this tool for diagnosis in my own, many years of practice.

Which Doctor?

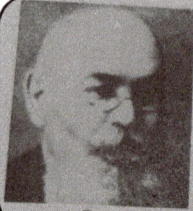

Dr. Von Peczely returned to Budapest in 1869, opened a homeopathic practice and soon gathered a large following. It was here that his only book, *Discoveries in the Realms of Nature and Art of Healing*, was published in 1880. For a time this work was conspicuously ignored by the scientific community and the press. Then in 1886, August Zoeppritz, editor of "Die Homeopatische Monatsblatter," published the news of von Peczely's discovery of iridology for all the world to see, while Dr. Emil Schlegel of Tubingen published a book on von Peczely's work, *The Eye-Diagnosis of I. V. Peczely*.

von Peczely

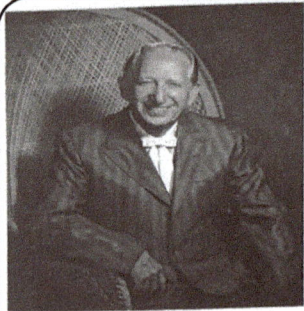

I Believe

I believe in iridology as the "eye" of the natural healing arts, the window through which the wholistic perspective on health becomes understandable.

I believe in iridology as a reliable means of assessing what is happening in the body. When we know what is happening in the body, we can choose the path to high-level wellness.

I believe in iridology as the analysis to use in any of the healing arts to monitor and evaluate how well a therapy is working.

I believe in iridology as the only analysis which reveals conditions before symptoms appear and shows abnormal conditions for which no symptoms will ever appear.

I believe in iridology as a wonderful means of demonstrating the rewards of choosing a healthy way of life, the ideal of preventive medicine.

I believe in iridology and nutrition as the twin guiding stars that will bring in a new profession equally uplifting for both doctor and patient.

I dedicate this book to my fellow iridologists and to iridology, the profession which I have been called to serve.

— Bernard Jensen
July 1982

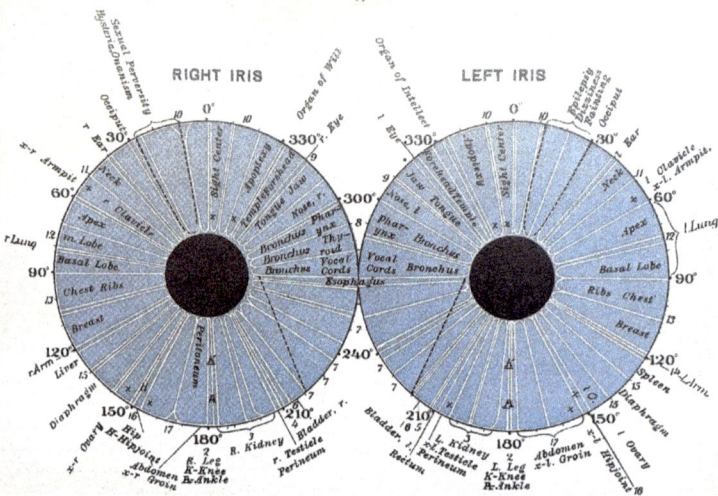

62

Bernard Jenson chart, a translation of the work of a Russian chart. This chart is still used today for iris diagnosis.

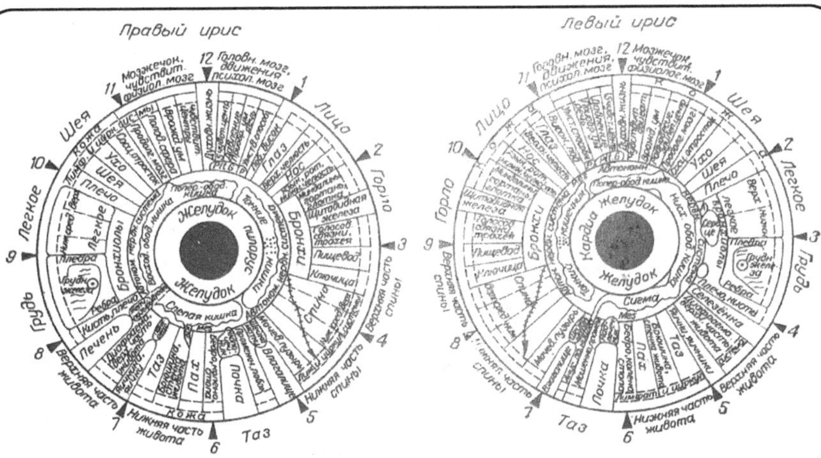

Рис. 1. Схема проекционных зон тела человека на радужной оболочке по Iensen.
Проекционные зоны «давление», «приобретенный ум», «речь», «умственные способности» соответствуют по топике лобной доле; «чувствительные центры», «духовная жизнь», «5 чувствительных центров»— теменной доле; «врожденный ум» — затылочной доле; «половая сфера», «равновесие», «эпилептический центр» — мозжечку.

Russian iris chart development based on the work of Dr. Bernard Jensen.

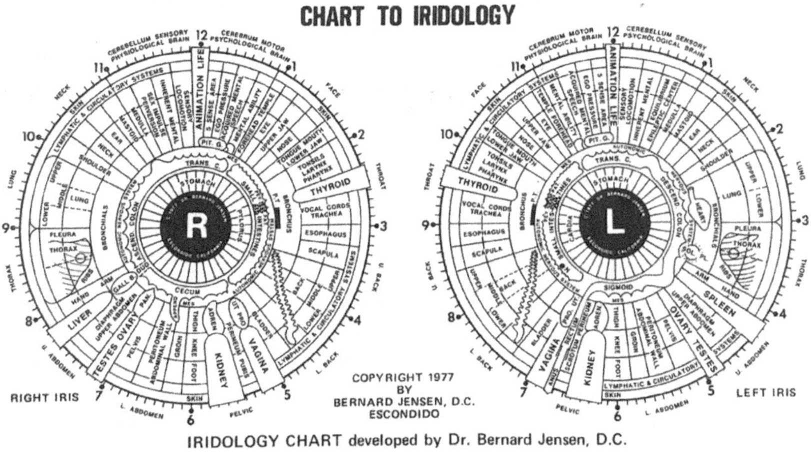

CHART TO IRIDOLOGY

COPYRIGHT 1977
BY
BERNARD JENSEN, D.C.
ESCONDIDO

RIGHT IRIS

LEFT IRIS

IRIDOLOGY CHART developed by Dr. Bernard Jensen, D.C.

Chart development and verification is a continuously ongoing research subject for Dr. Jensen.

How many times have you been to see the GP and said to them, "I'm so tired and exhausted and I don't know what's wrong with me. Please help," only to then have the GP do tests for your iron, your blood sugar, your thyroid function, your liver and kidney function, along with a full blood exam showing your red and white blood cells – perhaps even a test of your urine looking for infection?

You go back two weeks later for a follow-up appointment only to be told, "All your test results are normal. There is absolutely nothing wrong with you." What?! You leave the doctor's office feeling dejected and at a loss. You know it's not stress, and you're pretty sure you don't have a mental condition, so could it be all in your head? Maybe you start believing that it must be so?

YET, SOME PART OF YOU KNOWS YOU ARE NOT WELL AND IT IS NOT ALL IN YOUR HEAD.

Something is telling you to keep looking. We all have that inner voice, this intuition – even if at times we ignore it. Don't get me wrong, there can be *low* iron long before anaemia sets in, where you do not have enough red blood cells in your blood. And what about your B12 levels, vitamin D levels, folate, zinc, iodine, CoQ10 – just to name a few? Did your GP test for all these?

Did your GP ask whether you are you getting enough sleep? Whether you are drinking enough water? Or how much alcohol do you drink each week? Did they have time to check your blood pressure? How about, "Is there any stress in your life?" Too often the answer is no, they didn't ask and they didn't check because, unfortunately, doctors are not encouraged to spend time with their patients nor are they allowed to order extensive blood testing for each and every patient.

In the US, a patient often, if not always, pays for all their pathology testing, so if you are a low-income earner and can't afford to pay for blood testing or MRIs or ultrasounds or CT scans, then what diagnostic skills is your GP left with?

I recall a patient who had travelled five hours to see me at my clinic. She presented with extreme tiredness, very debilitating exhaustion. The doctors could find no explanation even though they had done several blood tests. But alas, no diagnosis could be made, and nothing was showing up in the tests they had done either. When she came to me, I took one look in her iris and found extremely clear signs of her thyroid being underactive. I asked whether her thyroid had been tested. She said no, as she had experienced no weight gain, no hair loss, and no other thyroid symptoms such as heart palpitations, intolerance to noise and motion – just this extreme tiredness. I said to her, "I'm sure it is your thyroid."

I prescribed my thyroid support formulas, asked her to get some fish and seaweed into her diet and put her on a vitamin D supplement. Vitamin D is very supportive to both thyroid and adrenal function. Of course, I also prescribed iodine (which Australian soil is very low in) and is so vital to thyroid function. I asked her to go back to her doctor in her local area and ask for thyroid blood tests, saying that her Naturopath says her thyroid needs further investigation.

The next thing I know, I received a letter from the GP thanking me for the recommendation and sending me my patient's thyroid results. It showed she had almost no T3 or T4 hormones, and her TSH hormone was extremely high in an effort to get her body to produce more. In layman's terms, her pituitary gland was working very hard making lots of thyroid-stimulating hormone (TSH) in order to get her thyroid gland to make more thyroid hormones, but it wasn't obliging, so she was running on empty and these hormones regulate calcium in your blood and female hormones in your body and even your immunity is affected by your thyroid hormones.

I was bowled over by the fact that this GP took the time to not only thank me, but send me her results. This co-operation was so amazing to me. Subsequently, this patient went onto make a full recovery with follow-up blood work showing marked improvement.

This is an example of where we could be working more closely with the family GPs and putting our skills together to achieve the best outcome for our shared patients. Without my iridology diagnostic tool searching out the cause of this patient's symptoms, I may have taken much longer, with much greater expense to the patient, trying to find an underlying cause for her existing malady.

Unfortunately, I have learned from the Naturopathic students seeking out clinical hours at my practice that they are being told iridology has no scientific evidence behind it, so it is no longer taught nor emphasised in their training. Yet this is a fundamental tool for discovery in my practice and has two centuries' worth of research papers, books, and experience, often written by medical doctors no less, who also used natural remedies and homeopathic approaches in their practice, combined with medical intervention to wonderful success with their sick, and often desperate, patients.

There has been an intentional plan to rid natural medicine from the medical community and training universities. Did you know, for example, The Alfred in Melbourne was once a homeopathic and osteopathic hospital working with medical practitioners to heal their patients right here in Melbourne, Australia? But that is a story for another day…

Iridology has now been replaced with psychology in Naturopathic course curriculums, and only "evidence-based medicine" is in the training. However, it seems to me the evidence has been cherry-picked and directed so as to weaken our Naturopathic courses and create a more clinical and pharmaceutical approach for the newly trained Naturopathic practitioner. Since when did psychology become a Naturopathic subject? Of course, we need rapport with our patients and kindness and compassion, but why cognitive behavioural therapy (a psychiatric technique, recently recommended in a recent naturopathic seminar)?

Caring for our patients and lifestyle changes have always been part of our knowledge and skill set. This is combined with the importance that we place on really *hearing* our patients, holding a safe space for them, believing in them when they tell you what *they* think could be their problem, and *not* evaluating or judging them for their story. This enables me as a doctor to better understand the full picture and evaluate what they are saying against my own skills and knowledge.

The trained psychologists I have seen doing any good at all are almost always using natural alternative approaches with their patients, along with referrals to Naturopaths or nutritionists, osteopaths, or chiropractors. Also teaching and recommending yoga and mindfulness, plus exercise – which again, is all in the realm of natural medicine.

Jumping back to iridology and the evidence and research, here is a recent article (August 2023) about the power of the eye to diagnose disease.

The Economist explains …

Can Parkinson's disease be detected with an eye exam?

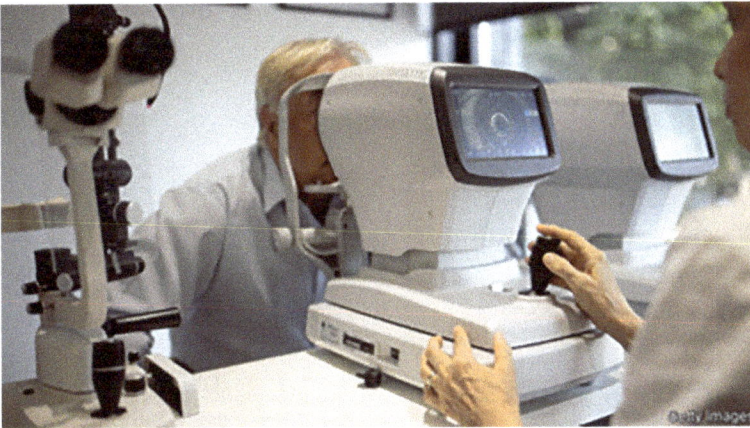

So-called "ocular biomarkers" may provide insights into brain health. It is often said that the eyes are the windows to the soul. Researchers hope that they might also be a window to the brain. Scientists wonder if eye scans could provide information about a wide range

of conditions, including ADHD, Alzheimer's disease, autism, schizophrenia and traumatic brain injury. They are already used to detect predispositions to physical-health problems like high blood pressure and diabetes. On August 21st, 2023, researchers at Moorfields Eye Hospital and University College at London's Institute of Ophthalmology published a paper in which they said they had identified markers of Parkinson's disease in the eye seven years before it would have been apparent using existing tests. How?

Changes in the eye, particularly the retina, sometimes appear to reflect changes in the brain. The retina is like a piece of wet tissue paper at the back of the eye that contains light-sensitive nerve cells in many distinct layers. It grows from the same tissue as the brain during embryonic development and is connected to the brain by the optic nerve. It thus shares many of the brain's characteristics. If a relationship between brain and retina were proved, it could be extremely useful: brains are difficult to study while their owners are alive. Eyes, on the other hand, are easy to scan in detail with equipment found in the average high-street optician's office. The technique in question is optical coherence tomography (OCT), a non-intrusive 3D scan that works by bouncing light waves across the eye and taking pictures of the retina and each of its layers, which are then mapped and measured.

The hunt for ocular "biomarkers" is a promising area of research. Pearse Keane, one of the authors of the recent Parkinson's study, says that scientists have known for more than a century that signs of diseases in the body can be detected with eye tests. Researchers hope that the proliferation of ocular pressure testing machines and advances in artificial intelligence will super charge their efforts. Ocular markers may one day help with efforts to prevent or slow the onset of degenerative diseases and even identify people suitable for trials of new drugs. Some envisage a day when they will guide personalised treatments. At the very least, this research is worth keeping an eye on!

End of article

I challenge this and say with iris diagnosis, the natural doctor can already plan individualised treatment plans NOW!

Preventative medicine is always more beneficial than waiting until the disease has taken hold of the body to such an advanced stage that only management is all one can hope for!

To finish this chapter, I wish to say one of the reasons for this book is to impart the knowledge that I see being lost in the teachings of today, not only in Naturopathy, but also in nursing, osteopathy, beauty therapy, and I suspect many other skill-based professions. I feel the quality of training and knowledge is getting lost in lieu of "evidence-based medicine" with double-blind trials all being done by pharmaceutical funded research institutes that are not only at the risk of being potentially biased but also have constant conflicts of interest.

A Cochrane Review done on many trials completed in the recent past often finds them lacking in ethics and in real-time evidence – and all too often conflicts of interest in the researchers themselves compromising the impartiality of the outcome!

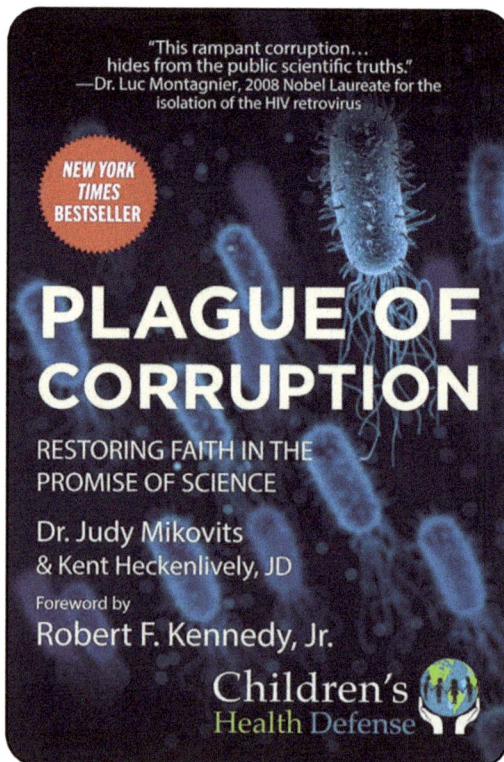

For more evidence of unethical behaviour in medicine, see this book.

When I did my double degrees, there were 14 written exams a year; 16 essays per year; and 500 hours of clinic: hands-on work with patients; as well as practical examinations showing the instructors how we massaged; how we did lymphatic drainage; how we did manipulations; and how we taught therapeutic exercises. We even made herbal medicines from scratch as fluid extracts. (I actually made all my individual herbal medicines from scratch in the first 10 years.)

I would love to see a college that was that thorough today in the quality control and examination of their student graduates in regards to their knowledge and application. How can online exams be trusted as a surefire way of testing a student's skill and comprehension?

Hats off to the Laws College of Naturopathy and Chiropractic where I was taught. Not only did we learn all that the Naturopathy colleges teach today, but we also did homeopathy, biochemistry of cells salts (low-dose minerals to assist the body with ailments), four years on nutrition with a great book, *The Composition and Facts About Food*, massage of various types, and water treatments like hot and cold compresses for pain and so much more. We even handwrote out our own herbal medicine books and submitted them to the dean of our college.

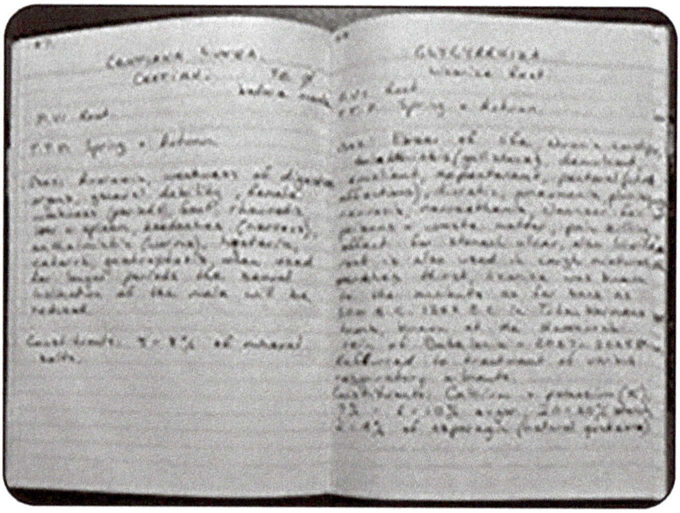

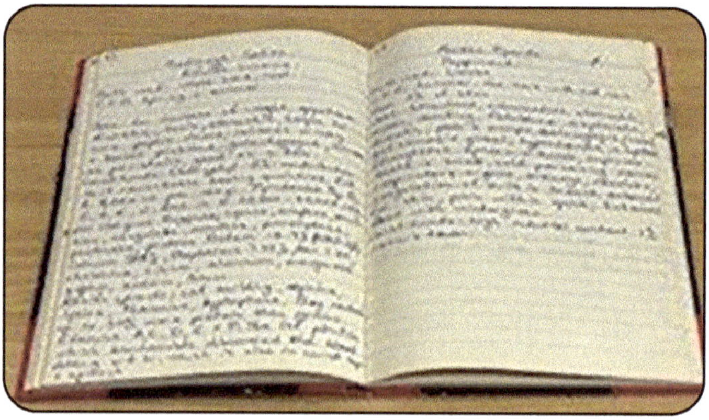

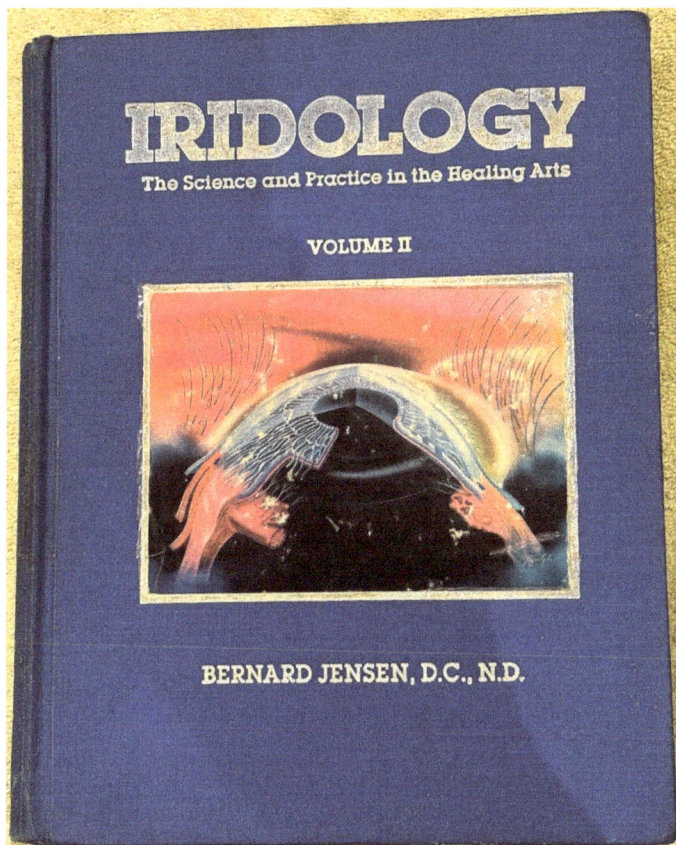

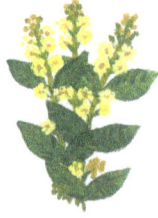

4

Alternatives To Medicating Your Child

For this chapter, let me start with a recollection of one of my daughter's experiences. She is eight-and-a-half months pregnant. She is enormous, and her baby is breach with the cord around the neck.

My daughter is told she has to have a cesarean section. She cries for a week as she had really wanted a natural birth. She herself was a home-birth baby with no drugs and experienced a very peaceful arrival. I reassured her and her husband that I would be there to support her fully.

Time moves on, and she has had enough of carrying such an enormous baby weight. She suffers hyperemesis, a severe form of morning sickness, which runs through the females in our family line.

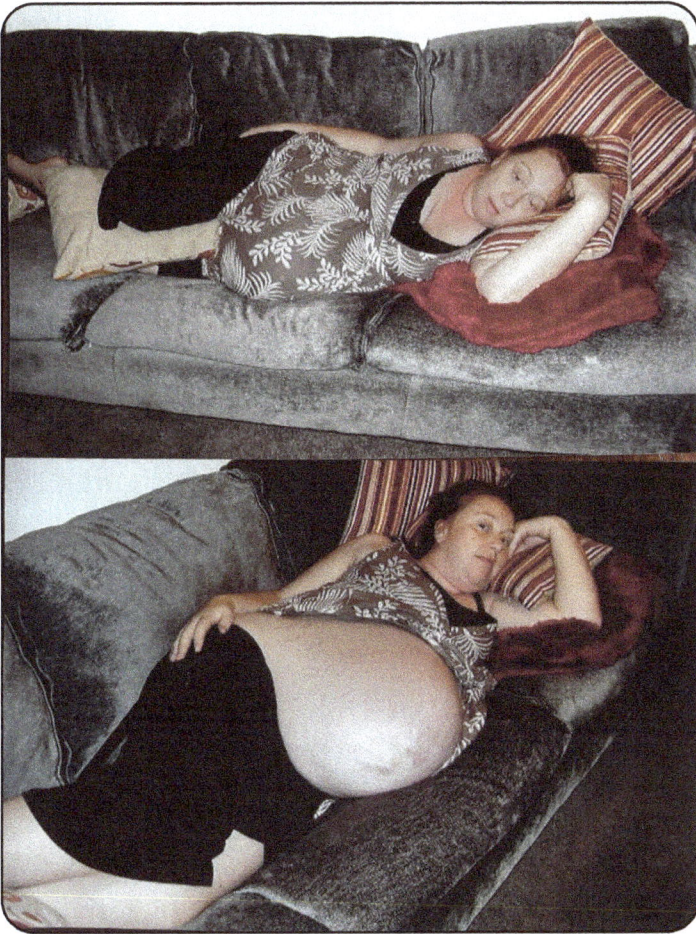

I decided to give her a homeopathic called caulophyllum to bring on the labour, as there was no hospital that had a bed for a pre-planned cesarean section any time soon in the whole of Melbourne (only beds for emergency cesareans).

She is by now dehydrated, exhausted, has been hospitalised during this pregnancy already and put on a drip to rehydrate her twice. She begs for my help to bring on her labour.

Within four hours of starting the homeopathic medicine, she was in labour. So off we went to the hospital, and an emergency cesarean section was undertaken. This was the first time my daughter had ever been in a hospital for any surgery, and after the operation, I went with her newborn baby, and my daughter was taken away with her husband by her side. They were unfortunately separated at birth, mother and baby.

I went to find her little one, my granddaughter. Here she was in a room, far away from her mother, in a humidity crib, all alone, with bright lights beaming down on her face, and screaming and sobbing uncontrollably. I immediately found something to put over her crib to dull the brightness. I opened up the side vent and put my hand in to hold her little waving arm, only to find her so hot she had perspiration dripping down her baby forehead. I quickly opened both sides of the closed-in crib to let some more air in so that she could breathe and cool down.

I then noticed her foot was blue: the name tag had been attached so tightly that it was cutting off her circulation to the foot. I ran to find a nurse to get it taken off, reassuring the little one that I would be back soon.

In the meantime, my daughter was experiencing severe itching all over her body, literally driving her mad. As it turned out, she was reacting to both the morphine and Panadol. The doctor came in and asked her, "Didn't you know you were allergic to these drugs?"

My daughter answers, "I have never had any drugs."

"Not even Panadol?" asks the doctor.

"No," my daughter says.

"Then what do you do if you need painkillers?"

"My mum is a Naturopath, so we just use natural medicines for pain if need be."

The doctor is shocked and says, "What, you have never even had a Panadol in your whole life?"

No, she had never had a Panadol.

Despite her severe allergic reaction to chemical-based drugs, had it not been for medical doctors that day, my daughter would never have had a baby safely. As it turns out, her uterus is heart-shaped and all three of her babies were breach, preferring to have feet down as their heads did not fit comfortably the other way around. On top of this, all her babies were huge, with short cords wrapped around their necks: 10lb (4.54kg), 11lb (4.99kg), and 13lb (5.90kg), respectively. So thank goodness for medical intervention in times like these.

There is definitely a place for all medical doctors and practitioners of the various kinds in this world.

Over the years, I have seen a lot of very sick children and there are times when medical intervention is lifesaving. However, there are many times where medical surgery or medical intervention is used when it could have been completely averted and is unnecessary.

I myself have assisted a lot of children over the years that were booked in for surgeries such as grommets, tonsillectomies, or adenoid removal, to become completely well without such – even things like jaw surgeries, nasal drilling, and pelvic intervention with casts on their lower body. I have lost count of the number of children, but it would be in the hundreds now that have not needed invasive medical intervention when it was recommended.

Children, in my opinion, respond very quickly and easily to homeopathic and herbal medicines, such as natural antibiotics, along with dietary changes to assist their conditions. Physical therapies, for example, massage, lymphatic drainage, spinal, ligaments and muscles realignment, therapeutic exercises, and even Bowen therapy… all can be life-changing for a child. And is very gentle!

VERTEBRAL SUBLUXATION AND NERVE CHART

"The nervous system controls and coordinates all organs and structure of the human body." (Gray's Anatomy, 29th Ed; page 4) Misalignment of spinal vertebrae and discs may cause irritation to the nervous system which could affect the structures, organs, and functions listed under "areas" and the "possible symptoms" that are associated with malfunctions of the areas noted.

Vertebrae	Areas & Parts of Body	Possible symptoms
C1	Blood supply to the head, pituitary gland scalp, bones of the face, brain, inner and middle ear, sympathetic nervous system.	❑ Headaches ❑ nervousness ❑ insomnia ❑ head colds ❑ high blood pressure ❑ migraine headaches ❑ nervous breakdowns ❑ amnesia ❑ chronic tiredness ❑ dizziness
C2	Eyes, optic nerves, auditory nerves, sinuses, mastoid bones, tongue, forehead.	❑ Sinus trouble ❑ allergies ❑ pain around the eyes ❑ earache ❑ fainting spells ❑ certain cases of blindness ❑ crossed eyes ❑ deafness
C3	Cheeks, outer ear, face bones, teeth, trifacial nerve.	❑ Neuralgia ❑ neuritis ❑ acne or pimples ❑ eczema
C4	Nose, lips, mouth, eustachian tube.	❑ Hay fever ❑ runny nose ❑ hearing loss ❑ adenoids
C5	Vocal cords, neck glands, pharynx.	❑ Laryngitis ❑ hoarseness ❑ throat conditions such as sore throat or quinsy
C6	Neck muscle, shoulders, tonsils.	❑ Stiff neck ❑ pain in upper arm ❑ tonsillitis ❑ chronic cough ❑ croup
C7	Thyroid gland, bursae in the shoulders, elbows.	❑ Bursitis ❑ colds ❑ thyroid conditions
T1	Arms from the elbows down, including hands, wrists, and fingers, esophagus and trachea.	❑ Asthma ❑ cough ❑ difficult breathing ❑ shortness of breath ❑ pain in lower arms and hands
T2	Hear, including its valves and covering, coronary arteries.	❑ Functional heart conditions and certain chest conditions
T3	Lungs, bronchial tubes, pleura, chest, breast.	❑ Bronchitis ❑ pleurisy ❑ pneumonia ❑ congestion ❑ influenza
T4	Gallbladder, common duct.	❑ Gallbladder conditions ❑ jaundice ❑ shingles
T5	Liver, solar plexus, circulation (general).	❑ Liver conditions ❑ fevers ❑ blood pressure problems ❑ poor circulation ❑ arthritis
T6	Stomach.	❑ Stomach troubles including ❑ nervous stomach ❑ indigestion ❑ heartburn ❑ dyspepsia ❑
T7	Pancreas, duodenum.	❑ Ulcers ❑ gastritis
T8	Spleen.	❑ Lowered resistance
T9	Adrenal and suprarenal glands.	❑ Allergies ❑ hives
T10	Kidneys.	❑ Kidney troubles ❑ hardening of the arteries ❑ chronic tiredness ❑ nephritis ❑ pyelitis
T11	Kidneys, ureters.	❑ Skin conditions such as acne ❑ pimples ❑ eczema ❑ boils
T12	Small intestines, lymph circulation.	❑ Rheumatism ❑ gas pains ❑ certain types of sterility
L1	Large intestines, inguinal rings.	❑ Constipation ❑ colitis ❑ dysentery ❑ diarrhea ❑ some ruptures or hernias ❑
L2	Appendix, abdomen, upper leg.	❑ Cramps ❑ difficult breathing ❑ minor varicoses veins
L3	Sex organs, uterus, bladder, knees.	❑ Bladder troubles ❑ menstrual troubles such as painful or irregular periods ❑ miscarriages ❑ bed wetting ❑ impotency ❑ change of life symptoms ❑ many knee pains
L4	Prostate gland, muscles of the lower Back, sciatic nerve.	❑ Sciatica ❑ lumbago ❑ difficult painful or too frequent urination ❑ backaches
L5	Lower legs, ankles, feet.	❑ Poor circulation in the legs ❑ swollen ankles ❑ weak ankles and arches ❑ cold feet ❑ weakness in the legs ❑ leg cramps
SACRUM	Hip bones, buttocks.	❑ Sacroiliac conditions ❑ spinal curvatures
COCCYX	Rectum, anus.	❑ Hemorrhoids (piles) ❑ pruritus (itching) ❑ pain at end of spine on sitting

ATLAS
AXIS
CERVICAL SPINE
1st THORACIC
THORACIC SPINE
1st LUMBAR
LUMBAR SPINE
SACRUM & COCCYX

NECK REGION
MID-BACK
LOW-BACK
PELVIS

See RESOURCE 4: Bowen Therapy

I have become very concerned with the labelling and medicating of our young children these days. As soon as a child is not listening, is running around too much for adults to cope with, or making too much noise and demonstrating their emotions, they are very quickly sent to a paediatrician or child psychiatrist.

From what I have been told by parents coming in with medicated children, it was only a five- or ten-minute consultation, and they were often told their child has some sort of disability resulting in poor behaviour or poor learning ability and they walk out with a script for an amphetamine-based drug to give to their child.

In many cases, it is my belief that so many of these children are just **unwell** and are in need of either better parenting skills, better teaching skills, less screen time (which is very introverting for a child), and much better nutrition, correction of vitamin or mineral deficiencies and treatment for food and environmental intolerances, along with more sleep. In one case in my practice it was the child's eyesight which was the issue, not ADHD as the parents were told.

This labelling of children can so easily happen.

The following example is something that occurred in my own practice. The phone rang at the clinic and one of my daughters – all grown up by now – answered the phone for the receptionist. On the other end of the line was a mother that wanted to book her son in for a consultation with one of our Naturopaths. She said to my daughter, "I'm sure that my son has ADHD." My daughter, having been brought up on natural foods and natural medicines her whole life said, "What makes you think that?" The mother says, "I just picked him up from kindergarten, and the teacher told me he was aggressive to some of the other kids, biting them, and that he would not settle down. He was being very hyperactive all morning."

My daughter, in her wisdom, asked, "What did your son have for breakfast today?" The mother then admitted that they were running late, so they stopped at a fast-food drive-in and got a burger and caffeinated soft drink for him. My daughter then kindly said, "Did you ever think his behaviour today might have something to do with the sugar, processed food, and caffeine in the breakfast he had?" The mother, bless her soul, says, "Do you really think what he ate had something to do with his behaviour today?" Of course, she booked him in to see one of our practitioners immediately.

This story serves to demonstrate that this child's mother had no idea of the concept of what we eat can and does influence our moods, behaviours, and/or sleep patterns. Had she gone to her GP, he would likely have given a referral for the child to get tested, and before too long, this child could have been put on unnecessary medication, with all their potential side-effects.

I have seen this happen more times than I can count. Just ask any kindergarten or primary school teacher how many children in their class are medicated these days. You'll be shocked at their answer.

See RESOURCE 5: Depression, Anxiety and Insomnia

Dr Mark Hyman spoke on a Tucker Carlson podcast 'Everything you're eating is toxic, and big Pharma likes it that way'. This all about sugar and the restriction of such from the diet making dramatic changes to autism, ADHD, learning disabilities, and even violence. He mentions in PubMed you can find research that has been done regarding this. He speaks of the diabetes in children being caused by sugar. He has created a foundation for functional health to assist Americans to turn this health disease around completely with diet and exercise alone.

You can watch free videos and seek out references here on www.cchr.or.au

In addition to these meds being prescribed often unnecessarily, some children can experience insomnia and anxiety from the medication itself, and if this goes on long enough, they can then develop depression.

As a side note, I have noticed that mothers on antidepressants while pregnant often have newborns that do not sleep. This will most likely be a direct result of selective serotonin reuptake inhibitors (SSRIs) affecting the neurotransmitter development of that forming baby in utero. This is my educated opinion only, for as far as I am aware, there have been no long-term independent studies done on the side-effects of the offspring of these women on psychological medications, while pregnant.

What I have found with a number of these manic and hard to handle children being labelled ADD, ADHD, hyperactive, or having learning processing disorders, is they just can't concentrate due to a diet full of processed *wheat*, which has been grown to produce high starch. The wheat is sprayed with a pesticide before it is planted which acts as a hormone disrupter to the human body. This GMO (genetically modified) crop creates blood sugar spikes so high that it is akin to giving your child a high sugar chocolate bar for breakfast before school each day. Processed foods with hidden sugars and carbs will do the same thing. This is most of your breakfast cereals being sold in your local supermarket today!

Alternatively, if you give these children a diet full of fresh organic fruits and vegetables with non-wheat whole grains and hormone-free chicken, grass-fed meats and wild-caught fish, you begin to see a very different child.

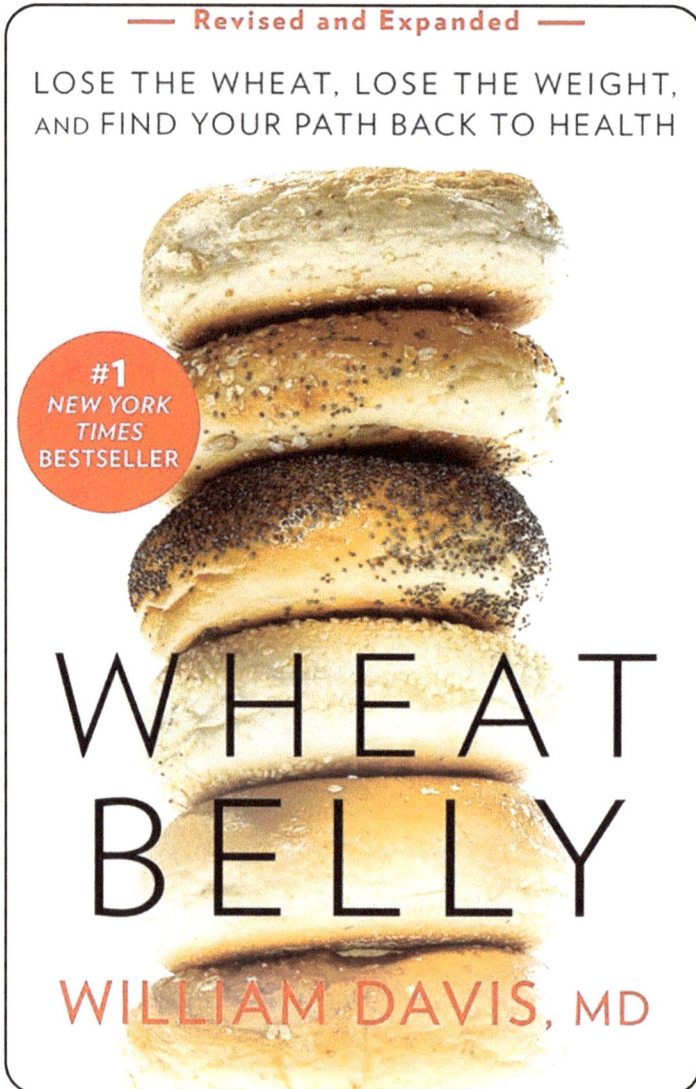

— Revised and Expanded —

LOSE THE WHEAT, LOSE THE WEIGHT, AND FIND YOUR PATH BACK TO HEALTH

#1 NEW YORK TIMES BESTSELLER

WHEAT BELLY

WILLIAM DAVIS, MD

So many of my patients over the years have reported that they can eat wheat in Italy or France, but not the US, Australia, New Zealand, or Canada. In these latter countries, they experience bloating, sleepiness after eating – caused by drops in their blood sugar after consumption – chronic tiredness, stomach cramps, and even eczema or dermatitis flare-ups. But they experience none of these symptoms if they eat the wheat in the European countries where it has been left untouched for hundreds of years.

A diet avoiding wheat, artificial colours (especially red colouring) and flavours, preservatives, MSG (often in stock cubes and instant noodles), along with avoiding concentrated processed sugars, soft drinks or sodas, is essential for children with both learning and behavioural difficulties.

All of these above processed foods contain chemicals within them affecting the insulin levels of a child dramatically, which in turn causes their blood sugar level to rise from the processed carbs or sugars. We then see a sudden subsequent drop in their blood sugar levels, causing the attendant child to melt down, fly into a rage, or fall into a dramatic crying mess on the floor (as if you just murdered their favourite pet but all you did was say "time for bed")!

Once the insulin and adrenal gland response sets in, this extreme fluctuation of blood sugar causes the child to experience a rollercoaster effect, resulting in a feeling of anxiety, weakness, and teariness, even a sullen disposition. The child may experience constant emotional meltdowns, throwing themselves on the floor in a mountain of tears very easily, or perhaps it is more of a brain fog and vagueness manifesting as lack of concentration.

You may have seen or know the child who always seems to be off with the fairies and not quite all there, with you. It is like no one is home in these children and they can't be reasoned with. (This is typical of someone on street drugs or alcohol as well.). They are in their own world and not interested in their present surroundings. They may become very aggressive for not getting their own way and feel they are being interrupted by normal life events or other actions an adult wants a child to do.

To engage a child experiencing this is tough on both teachers and parents alike, so they are given amphetamine class of drugs in order to wake them up artificially and get them to be present all the while, at the same time, the drug, being so strong on their bodies, they are somewhat sedated, making them more controllable and malleable for both parents and teachers. If these doctors were to use sedatives only, such as valium, these children would be falling asleep in class, hence the choice of an amphetamine class of drug is used instead.

There is research coming out now about the gut microbiome and chronic disease being linked to antibiotic use in children. One such article found in PubMed (published in 2021) called 'Association between antibiotics and gut microbiome dysbiosis in children: systematic review and meta-analysis' outlines this exact statement. This gut flora, or lack thereof, influences a child's immune response, potentially leading to many food intolerances, environmental sensitivities, and imbalances in the child's neurotransmitters, some of which rely on gut health, to be produced. This means serotonin, the calming hormone, or even dopamine, the happy hormone, and melatonin, the sleep hormone, all can be adversely affected by the lack of enough diverse gut flora, leading then to sleep disturbances, anxiety, or dramatic changes in the child's general behaviour.

Such natural medicines as probiotics, magnesium, activated B vitamins, vitamin D, iron plus herbs like chamomile for calming, *Melissa officinalis* (lemon balm) for anxiety, *Ziziphus spinosa* (Chinese herb) for sleep and even homeopathic melatonin or actual melatonin from the pharmacy can assist your child to sleep more deeply and enough. All of these above natural medicines assist in balancing the child's nervous system, immune system, neurotransmitter system, and gut microbiome without risk of addiction or side-effects.

So many young ones are not getting the 10 to 12 hours of sleep their bodies need while growing so quickly, often leading to nervous-system exhaustion in these children. The natural medicines give the child a chance to balance themselves and optimise the epigenetic (outside influences on the body) response in their growing bodies and to the environment.

With such a heavy push on vaccines and penalties now imposed by governments if your child does not receive the required 54 vaccines by the age of four years old, it is now implanting the belief a child doesn't have a chance of surviving without these vaccines, all the while negating the fact that a child does have its own innate and strong immune system to assist in their recovery if they do get measles, whooping cough, influenza virus, or some other childhood virus or infection. You can refer to the National Immunisation schedule (childhood) to confirm the number of recommended vaccines these days.

When a child is born vaginally, coming through the birth canal, it exposes them to a number of beneficial bacteria and microbiome to assist their immune development.

Furthermore, the colostrum secreted at the beginning of breastfeeding, prior to mother's milk coming in, is full of antibodies the mother has developed in her life which, in turn, affords the child's body with a headstart in natural immunity.

As the first months of growth occur, the child's body picks up various bacteria, viruses, and toxins, all of which start to activate the child's natural immune defences that then produce more of their own antibodies. This is their innate immune defence system at work which protects against infections, but also strengthens their natural killer cells, so if they *do* get so sick they *can* recover.

If your child has a happy home life and is getting good sleep, good food, and is well hydrated with pure water, this is often the best defence you can give your child when they are growing up. One of the excellent natural immune medicines I have in the clinic is a colostrum-based formula, with probiotics, to improve the immunity of a bottle-fed baby whose mother did not have the option of breastfeeding their baby.

So let the dog lick their face, let them play in the dirt: all this attention on disinfecting everything in sight in the home, kindergarten, and school is preventing their natural immunity from developing.

I also don't believe in spoiling a child with love, pour it on and they will blossom under your care and guidance.

In hospitals now, I have become aware through direct experience, women are being told NOT to give a newborn baby any water. Our bodies are made up of 70% water. As long as the water is pure and boiled to remove any bad bacteria, it is very safe to give a newborn some water and, in some cases, important to introduce water at a young age. Breastmilk is naturally very sweet, so it is important to introduce babies to something that is not so sweet early to assist in developing their sense of taste. In the hot summer, a baby may need water, but not so much in the cold winter.

When I went to hospital to visit my first grandchild, she was only a day old and my daughter's milk had not yet come in. The baby was crying and crying when I got there, and I soon found out this had been going on for hours. My daughter was distressed, and the nurses kept saying to her that, "You need to rest, and we will take care of your baby in the nursery." She couldn't get up or walk as she had just had a cesarean section. A mother knows her baby's cry and she kept asking them to look after her baby or bring her back to her. This was not happening.

When I got there, the nurses were understaffed and run off their feet. They didn't have the time to even answer the mother's call button. I went to get the baby, and her lips were very dried up, almost cracking. The ward was very hot, and she was a big baby. I asked the nurse for a bottle so I could give the baby some boiled water. No, they would not allow that anymore, I was told!

Seeing how dehydrated the newborn looked, I boiled some water, cooled it down, put it into a medicine glass, and gave the baby a drink. She guzzled down the full 40mls that I had put in the medicine glass and promptly went straight off to sleep. My daughter was so relieved and could now sleep herself. I promised to stay and look after her little one so she could get some well-deserved rest.

I think each case needs to be evaluated in its own right against these policies that are introduced carte blanche into hospitals. They are not always suitable to each and every case, and it is necessary for some degree of human judgement to enter into different situations.

When your child is sick, sometimes it is wise to go straight to a hospital or a medical doctor, but there are times where allowing your child to go through a cough, a cold, diarrhoea, or a high fever is part and parcel of that child's body developing their own strength of immunity, so the next time they *are* exposed to croup or a flu, their innate immunity can fight it and they can get better quickly.

A homeopathic first-aid kit is often handy to have along with vitamin C, vitamin D and zinc (which Australian soil is very deficient in), some herbal cough mixture, and perhaps my infection fighter. (See recipes in the Resources section at the end of this book.) Or perhaps your child's body could benefit from a herbal natural antibiotic? Such as olive leaf extract, readily available in health food stores and some pharmacies.

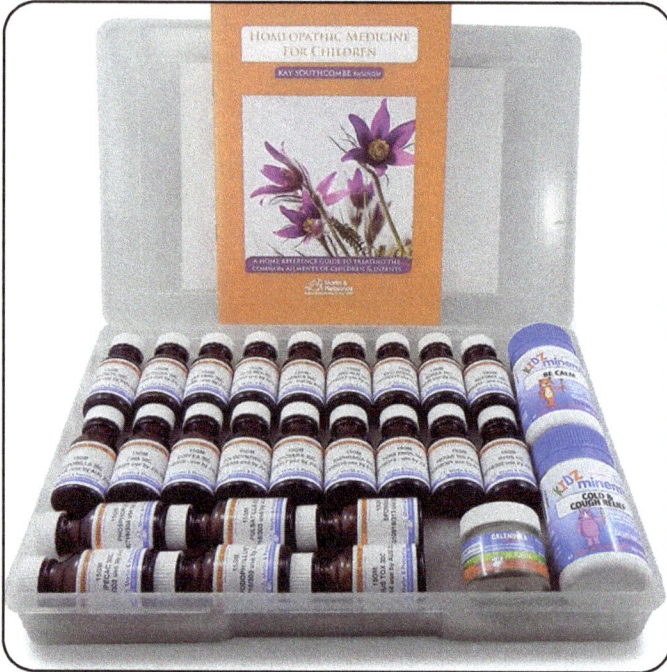

As my girls were growing up, there was a case of measles that went through the primary school they both attended. There were approximately 50 children in that school: children that *were* vaccinated against the measles; children that had had *homeopathic prophylactic medicines for* childhood measles; children that were not vaccinated at all – it was a real cross-section.

This particular strain of measles was very strong, and almost all the kids in that school caught this particular case, my girls included, and this is what I saw: the medically vaccinated kids got really sick; my girls who were not vaccinated got mildly sick but were back at school fairly quickly; and the homeopathic vaccinated children varied, some were really sick and others not so sick.

My conclusion to this observation was that it does not seem to matter whether your child is vaccinated or not, they can still get sick. What seems to matter the most, however, is how nutritionally balanced is the child? How strong is that child's immunity? How strong is that child's constitution? In other words, how strong is their genetic or inherited health from their parents, grandparents, and great-grandparents? How happy and secure is that child in their home and school? All these factors play, in my opinion, a very large part in the health and longevity of each and every child when it comes to health and wellbeing.

One other story that comes to mind: I had been in practice about 15 years when one of my Naturopaths who had a baby boy had chosen not to vaccinate him. He contracted whooping cough, and he was taken to the Royal Children's Hospital in Melbourne. I went to see him and my colleague. She felt so guilty for not vaccinating. She was made to feel this way by the attending nurses and doctor. I arrived to find ten babies in the ward all with whooping cough, the other nine *were* medically vaccinated. So out of ten, one was not medically vaccinated, but the other nine were. I believe this ratio alleviated some of my colleague's guilt.

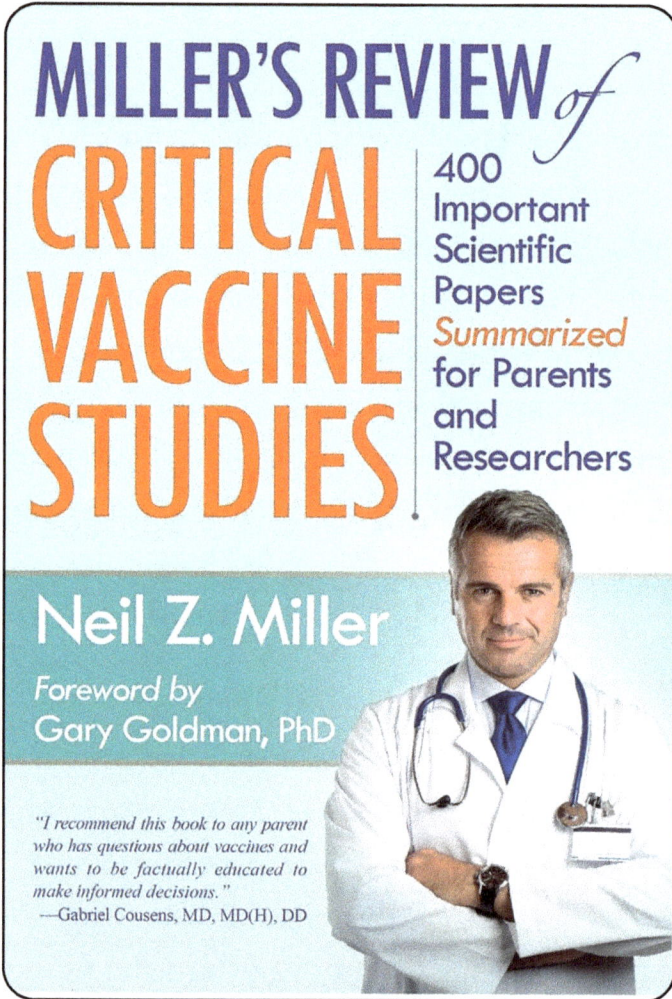

These true-life experiences go a long way toward my conclusion, which is that I don't think anything is foolproof, meaning nothing can be 100% guaranteed when it comes to vaccinations protecting your child from the common childhood diseases!

The best approach you can adopt for your child's health is to make sure they are eating a nutritionally balanced diet with nutrient-dense organic food, well slept, and drinking sufficient good-quality purified water, that they are physically active, and are surrounded by a loving family who care and supports them. Coincidentally, these ideas hark back to my second chapter, where I discussed the five laws of nature, which are the underlying principles of Naturopathy and the alternative medicine approach to wellness.

For children with coughs and colds, I recommend:

- Vitamin C, powder or chewable, with bioflavonoids, which enhance the action of this vitamin internally. 500 to 1000mg two to three times a day for young children.
- Vitamin D, which is not only immune boosting but is also antiviral. 2000 to 3000 IU up to twice a day. This dose only while sick.
- Zinc, up to 30 mg per day for a sick child, and 11mg as a maintenance dose – in winter months especially.
- Herbs such as olive leaf extract, a natural antibiotic, propolis, astragalus, echineaca, and goldenseal, to name a few.

- There are herbal formulas that, if added to pure vegetable glycerine, will sweeten the herbs to be given to children as a cough elixir as well.

See RESOURCE 6: Natural Antibiotics

Vitamin A is very important for preventing asthma, lung, and bronchial weaknesses in children. Short-term, high doses of vitamin A have long been known to bring about complete recovery for croup, asthma, and bronchiolitis sufferers. This vitamin is essential in the repair of inflamed mucous membranes, which is the lining of our nose, throat, bronchus, bronchioles, and lungs. I also recommend essential oils, such as Easy Air from the Dōterra range, to be used as a chest rub and to diffuse by the child's bed overnight.

I recall one such success story of an eight-month-old baby girl with a malignant tumour of the eye. She was undergoing chemotherapy, thereby having her white blood cells drastically compromised, which is the case with all chemotherapy. She then contracted a chest infection with a severe cough. The medical antibiotics were not helping. She was struggling to breathe, so in a phone consultation with her mother, I recommended her to rub the essential oils onto her chest, on her pillow, and to be diffused. The parents reported a marked recovery within three days just doing this alone. Of course, I was over the moon for this little one.

I have had my share of treating babies with cancer, while under the care of Royal Children's Hospital protocols, all of whom have gone on to be survivors and thriving with full lives, free of pain and suffering, which they all once knew. I'll go into more detail in my cancer chapter later in this book.

Over the years, I have treated a lot of extremely young babies, many of whom I found can be intolerant to their mother's breast milk or their baby formula, sometimes vomiting up a lot of their milk after feeding. They are also not sleeping well, often due to their stomach pains, wind, and restlessness. In this case, I look for lactose intolerance and/or casein intolerance (the protein in all animal breast milk), often pointing to the need for beneficial probiotic bacteria to assist their digestion in the production of these needed enzymes. These enzymes can then break down the lactose and proteins found in the breast milk or baby formulas.

In such a case, giving my herbal colic drops of dill, probiotics for babies or homeopathic medicines for colic will not be enough, so I then recommend the NAET treatment that I have mentioned earlier.

NAET is a treatment based on the principles of acupuncture and Chinese Medicine philosophy, and it incorporates homeopathic glass vials, with minute doses of casein or lactose or the breast milk or formula held within each vial. We place these vials onto the baby's body, usually in their socks or booties against their skin, while the mother holds her baby, and we use mum for the muscle response testing. This is called surrogate muscle testing, and it is used for testing sensitivities by muscle strength also known as neurosensitivity testing.

We then treat for these sensitives by stimulating acupressure points down the spine of the baby. A gentle tapping action begins the reset of the child's nervous and immune systems, allowing their body to clear away any aberrated or unwanted patterns in these systems that is the cause of their reaction to the breast milk or formula ingredients.

This NAET treatment then allows their body to absorb and process the lactose or casein or lactic acid contained within the breast milk or baby formula. The child then returns to the clinic to have these vials of homeopathic substances retested to make sure their little bodies are now able to tolerate and digest their food. Of course, we are also very interested to hear how well this baby is doing in regards to their symptoms. Has the vomiting stopped? Are they sleeping better? Are their colic pains abating?

Ayla Abou-Sinna 2-year-old child-Success Story

Our daughter's Journey:

When Ayla was born, we had no idea about wholistic health and the health conditions and treatments surrounding it. After birth, she had what we thought was general colic and fussiness. As she grew older, she started to develop further symptoms of fussiness and irritability. At 4 months old, we started to notice skin irritation that looked like eczema. It proceeded to worsen over the weeks and months, with some severe fluctuations in between. We sought the help of every modern medicine doctor, general practitioners and specialists, and we were constantly told that it was based on allergies and to use steroid treatment and to rely on "chance" for a cure. For months and months, after countless visits and money spent, we were in a constant circle with no light in sight.

That was until we stumbled across Dr Nerida James' clinic. We found her after Google searching healing cream for eczema, which led us to Dr Nerida's Skin Aid which helped greatly!

After our first visit with Dr Nerida, she told us what no other doctor had ever told us. Ayla can be helped! We were stunned and so excited at the possibility. Three months later and several NAET treatments for food and dust mite intolerances, Ayla's eczema had completely disappeared, her food allergies, which were partly anaphylactic, were gone and her overall bubbly personality has shone through.

We owe so much to Dr Nerida and her wonderful practice and we have gone on to recommend everyone we know to her for any health issues.

Kind regards,
Sylvia, Mother

I have found the NAET technique a very valuable tool as an adjunct to herbal medicine, homeopathic medicine, and nutritional medicine, along with dietary changes that we in Naturopathy are so passionate about. All of these approaches contribute greatly to improving your child's health, happiness and, most importantly, their emotional wellness.

I have seen countless mothers cry with relief in my clinic at how quickly their baby starts to sleep and then smile, after weeks, if not months, of rocking their crying little ones back and forth that could not sleep due to pain, suffering, and sometimes, even malnutrition. This help and gratitude from parents that I and many of my colleagues have experienced is what keeps us practising and working late into our years when many would have retired. I know the principal of my college kept practising even into her 90th year of life.

In this day and age, medicating children starts at birth and often continues through their childhood in the form of paracetamol, which lowers glutathione, hence lowering their immune system even further. Fifty-four vaccines are now injected by the time a child is four years old, including the prescription of multiple courses of antibiotics given for their coughs, colds, ear infections, and even viral infections.

Whilst there is truth in a child's immune system creating antibodies against different diseases introduced to their bodies through vaccines or through illness, where are the independent studies on the effects of the *chemicals* that have been added to these vaccines?

Such substances as:

a) Nano particles of aluminium (an adjunctive added) which crosses the blood brain barrier.

b) Benzoate (preservative added).

c) Polysorbate 80, another additive to vaccines.

d) Thimerosal (the mercury) a preservative in the flu vaccine.

All are injected into young babies and children.

Can anyone show me studies done on babies showing these chemicals are safe for newborns and young children?

Which Doctor?

Without these immunisation scheduled vaccinations being given, your children won't be allowed to attend preschool. Nor will you as the parents be entitled to your $5,000 child bonus from our government here in Australia. Just go to the vaccination schedule in our Australian government website to verify this statement.

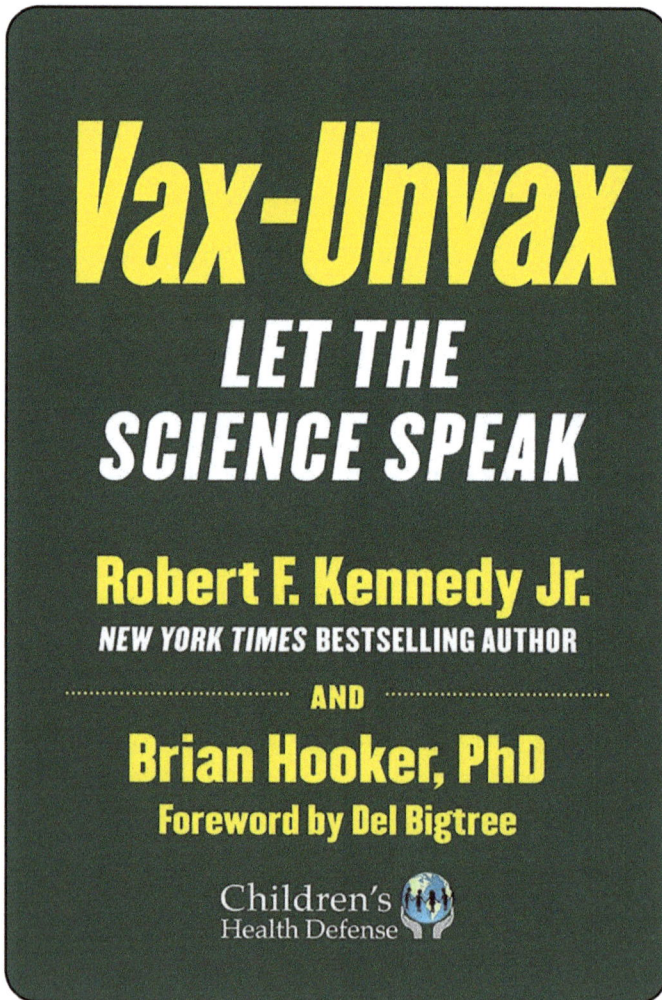

See RESOURCE 7: Pregnancy Birthing Kit

To finish this chapter, I have included here my homeopathic birthing kit to assist before, during, and after labour. This is for women wanting to naturally help their birthing process, minimise risk of intervention during such a natural and life changing experience as birth and babies.

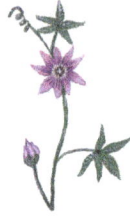

5

Hormone Balance

Puberty, Fertility, Contraception, Menopause, and Andropause (male menopause)

Over the many years in practice, I have seen patients with very severe hormone imbalances, both men and women, as well as young teenagers going through puberty.

Let's start with the young ones, typically anywhere between the ages of 10 to 17 years old. Do you remember that age? Sore breasts so tender you can't bare even a singlet to touch them. Emotions running wild and being so oversensitive that you find yourself slamming a door on your mum or dad over just being spoken to kindly. Crying hysterically over the girlfriend who betrayed you or your mate that asked the girl out that you liked with no consideration of your feelings.

Then to top it off, your skin starts to break out, it even feels sore to touch. It gets red and inflamed, which makes you not want to go out or even go to school. You feel like you look ridiculous. There is no hope. You segregate yourself. You feel a combination of shyness and anger. You constantly feel upset and overly self-conscious, so you try to cover up all of your insecurities by being angry and all this can make you very introverted...

This is a tough time for many teenagers! To make it worse, parents often overreact themselves to this behaviour, as it is all too close to their own behaviour as they were growing up. But of course, this is very much forgotten and pushed down in the memory of our parents.

Here is what I have found very helpful in such situations and are needed for the building blocks of hormones in adolescents:

- Calcium and magnesium – calms down the nervous system.

- Make sure they are getting enough sleep, even extra sleep.

- Activated B-Complex vitamins – supports the nervous system and assists in stabilising emotions. Also fantastic for memory, so needed in studies at school.

- Extra B1 – 100mg up to three times a day, especially for grief and emotional sensitivity.

- Evening primrose oil in capsule form or liquid (if they can't swallow capsules) up to 1000mg twice a day and premenstrual 2000mg twice a day (for girls) – needed to assist the body's manufacture of hormones, as is other natural oils like vitamin E.

- Blackcurrant seed oil is another good alternative to evening primrose oil and I often give this to blood type O patients as this is a super food for them according to the *Eat Right for Your Blood Type* book by Dr.Peter J. D'Adamo.

For girls, their body is making more hormones, which is why hair grows under the arms and around the pubic area. Their breasts start to grow, but very often I see not enough progesterone being made, giving rise to late onset of menstruation or periods that are very painful, irregular, and very heavy for the first day or so. A lot of the time, premenstrual tension is also way worse than should be experienced.

This low progesterone can also cause 'oestrogen dominance' and the young women can then experience weight gain because of this imbalance. Even endometriosis (an overgrowth of the cells inside the uterus escaping outside into the abdominal cavity) may occur.

Sometimes I have to add in herbal medicine to assist the hormone production, such as wild yam or chaste tree also known as *Vitex agnus-cactus*. I often recommend this along with zinc, false unicorn, blue cohosh, and dong quai: herbs which can boost this hormone production.

The GP's answer to the above for these young women is often *the pill*. In other words, their body is not making enough hormones, so they then prescribe artificial hormone replacement therapy which unfortunately can come with many attendant side-effects. Also, it is not addressing the low hormones or encouraging their own body to correct things! In fact, this just worsens the 'oestrogen dominance'.

See RESOURCE 8: Side-effects of the Contraceptive Pill

For the boys, puberty can cause them to be quick to anger, become more aggressive, restless, and rebellious. They just want to get out into the world and do stuff! Along with the above, they can also experience emotional reactions to their acne breakout and increased hormones…

In their case, I have often suggested young men take GABA powder at night, which modulates neurotransmitters and has a calming effect. I also recommend a lot of exercise and getting them into sports and games they can strive to win, be a team member and help them to feel they belong somewhere.

I also suggest using a lot of essential fatty acids which can be found in fish oils or algae, as these are oils high in omega 3,

6, and 9. These oils assist in making hormones and help with cognitive function and learning.

Zinc is also an important mineral because this aids in the treatment of acne and helps modulate and regulate their hormones – up to 30 mg twice daily and extra vitamin C is great in cleaning up their acne.

Now, for the next very important point both for acne and hormone balance, young people must be educated in the importance of good nutrition and which foods encourage hormone imbalances that lead to consequences such as acne.

Dairy products are terrible for encouraging acne. Cow's milk is full of sugar and fat that acne loves, and it congests the lymphatic system. There are also growth hormones in cow's milk to make baby calves grow big and fat; this too can have that effect on some young teenagers, thereby creating hormone imbalance.

Avoiding cane sugar is also recommended as this can be inflammatory and encourages the bacteria in acne to proliferate in the skin and the period pain in girls to become even worse.

If you search PubMed, you will find evidence of cutting out sugar thus improving behaviour, aggression, and oversensitive emotional reactions to life.

Next thing to watch out for is chicken and beef, both of which can be full of hormones given to the animal to increase their growth and weight, therefore making them more profitable at sale time. Did you know in chicken farms, baby chicks grow to full size in six weeks, but if left out in nature, it takes 18 to 20 weeks to grow a chicken to full size? This means three batches of chickens can grow in the time it would take one batch to grow naturally.

One of my patients many years ago got his chicken food analysed. My patient showed me the results sheet, which came back showing 36 different chemicals in the chicken food, many of which were antibiotics. These are used to stop the poor chickens from getting sick living locked up in a shed, crammed together so they can barely move, along with growth hormones and oestrogen to speed up the baby chicken's development.

In regards to beef, it is often stained with red colouring to make it look better, but this red dye is terrible for brain cells and like alcohol, can kill cells off. The cattle can also be given hormones to fatten them up for sale and are overfed corn to create more fat cells in the beef. This is your meat marbled with fat.

Last but not least is wheat, as mentioned in the above chapter: Australian wheat is bastardised. It creates a high glycemic spike in blood sugar, and that puts stress on the pancreas and adrenals whilst influencing hormone balance adversely. Plus, like sugar, wheat encourages acne to become worse.

I recommend severely hormone imbalanced teenagers to stop consuming so much dairy, concentrated sugars, hormone-fed meats, and processed white wheat. This can make a world of difference in a very short time to their skin and moods.

Combining the above education with herbs, vitamins, and minerals, subsequently leads to fast improvement in the hormone development of young teenagers. I have seen results such as greatly increased happiness and improved school performance, along with better energy and general wellbeing.

Fertility, contraception, and conception.

This is for women aged 20 to 48 years old. I have done extra study in this area of expertise and received a certificate in 'Natural Fertility Management'.

I had my first baby at 20 years old and it was the best thing I ever did, as I was young, full of energy, and pursuing my career. This idea that you can't have babies and have a career is a misleading one. I did both, and love my daughters dearly. I still would give my life for them. There is no end to a mother's lioness type protection for her children and her children's children.

Did you know at least 4 women in every 10 are experiencing miscarriages in this day and age as per published research article BMC Pregnancy and Childbirth on 22 Dec 2017 in PubMed? That's 43% miscarrying. Why?

I have had good success over the years in assisting both women and men with infertility to conceive their first child.

Here is what I have found:

1. There is a cause of miscarriage in women due to there being high DNA fragmentation of the *male sperm*. So guys, your body can be responsible for your partner's early pregnancy loss. So not only doing a sperm count but also getting a DNA fragmentation test done on your sperm may be important in resolving your partner's apparent infertility.

2. I have also found males with low sperm count or poor motility (swimmers) and high abnormal sperm in their test results, leading to infertility in women.

3. For women, I have found low progesterone as a leading cause of miscarriage. In this case, I would recommend such things as evening primrose oil twice a day to start with. This is one of the essential oils your body needs to

manufacture hormones, along with oils in your diet, such as olive oil, avocados, nuts, and seeds.

Then there are also herbs that assist your body to produce more progesterone, such as dong quai, blue cohosh, wild yam, chaste tree, and false unicorn. This is when I would advise my progesterone tonic two to three times a day, especially pre-menstrually.

4. For men, I recommend zinc, vitamin C, and the herb called *Tribulus terestris*, along with activated B vitamins and CoQ10 (ubiquinol).

5. Uterine and colon infections, such as the common *Candida albicans*, can alter the microbiome of the vagina and uterus, often causing acidity or excess alkalinity. These imbalances can create a high NK cell (natural killer cell) presence in the vagina and uterus. This, in turn, can cause the destruction of the partner's sperm. This can also be tested for by your fertility specialist.

If this is the case, we detox the woman's body by using antimicrobial herbs or antifungal or anti-parasitic herbs to kill off such things as *Streptococcus, Giardia, Candida albicans*, parasites, and/or amoebas, etc. It's also important to alkalise the body with minerals, along with probiotics, especially strains that are present in the vagina and those that help crowd out the excess bad bacteria. In other words, we need to restore the microbiome to a congenial state for fertility.

This is important for male fertility and applies to male sperm as well as the pH of the body and restoring their microbiome too.

Here, I like to use berberine herbs, pau d'arco, black walnut, cloves, *Artemisia annua*, oregano oil, thyme oil, and grapefruit seed extract to name a few. For the probiotics, I like to use Bifidobacterium strains and *Lactobacillus rhamnosus* and *Saccharomyces boulardi*. These are the good bacteria strains that especially inhabit the adverse bacteria in the vagina and reduce likelihood of thrush or other microbial infestations.

6. Lower back impingement can also be detrimental to fertility, especially of the third lumbar. This is where the blood and nerve supply come from to feed both the uterus and ovaries in females, or the prostate, testes, and genitalia in males. Massage and manipulation and trigger point therapy or Bowen therapy for lower-back issues can come into play here as well.

The importance of exercise also cannot be overstated in order to increase the blood flow to these organs and to increase the hormone production and get them flowing around the body. Exercise can also assist the lower back to stay aligned and mobile, once the bodywork has been done.

7. Lymphatic drainage can be another fantastic tool to assist fertility in both males and females. I especially like the German technique known as the Vodder method of manual lymph drainage.

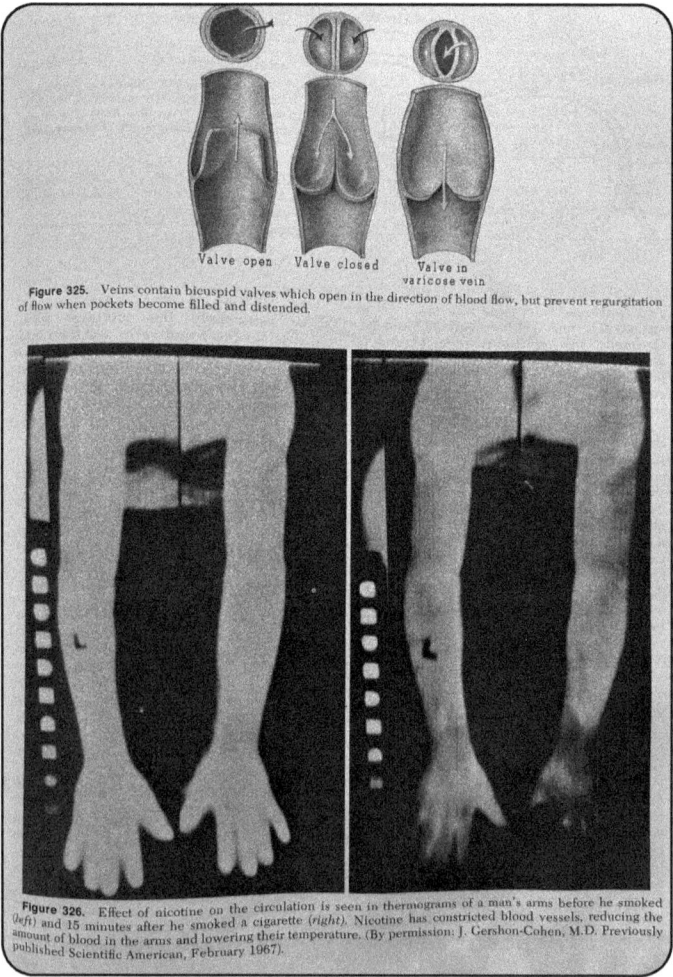

Valve open   Valve closed   Valve in varicose vein

Figure 325. Veins contain bicuspid valves which open in the direction of blood flow, but prevent regurgitation of flow when pockets become filled and distended.

Figure 326. Effect of nicotine on the circulation is seen in thermograms of a man's arms before he smoked (left) and 15 minutes after he smoked a cigarette (right). Nicotine has constricted blood vessels, reducing the amount of blood in the arms and lowering their temperature. (By permission: J. Gershon-Cohen, M.D. Previously published Scientific American, February 1967).

8. Cigarette smoking is extremely harmful to fertility because nicotine causes blood vessels to constrict, reducing the blood flow to the fertility organs. Any failure I have had in my practice with infertility cases is with males or females that can't stop smoking.

For those who are lucky enough to conceive and keep smoking, here is an article we were given in Naturopathic college called "Child Abuse: The Most Pervasive Way to Injure Your Child."

See RESOURCE 9: The Most Pervasive Form of Child Abuse

This sounds very alarming, doesn't it? But in a research trial, ultrasound was administered to a pregnant woman while she smoked a cigarette. It showed how the baby screwed up its little face in pain as she smoked and cut down the circulation (oxygen) to her baby momentarily while she was smoking. Imagine doing that to your baby 10 or 15 times a day while smoking each cigarette. Is it any wonder these babies are born smaller and often with lung and bronchial weaknesses?

9. Hormonal imbalances can also cause issues. After years and years on the pill, there can be oestrogen dominance

once a woman comes off the pill. This dominance can cause miscarriages.

In this case, it is about getting the liver to detox the excessive oestrogen and thereby balancing the hormonal cycle. The way to tell if you are balanced is to see how much premenstrual tension or symptoms you are experiencing. Do you have terrible breast tenderness or severe uterine cramps during your bleed? Or are you very teary and depressed before your cycle? Or are you extremely irritable and have headaches or migraines around period time? These are all indicators of hormonal imbalance, and to have a healthy uncomplicated pregnancy, you must balance those hormones first.

To help oestrogen dominance, I recommend DIM, an activated form of indole 3 carbinol, a substance from soya beans that assists your liver to clear the excessive oestrogen that can build up from taking the pill. Also, broccoli sprouts are great for helping the liver detox pathways, assisting oestrogen clearance. There are amino acids like methionine, along with activated B vitamins, that can also assist. These help the liver to metabolise these excess oestrogens and thereby reducing the risk of cancers that are oestrogen fed.

To finish this section on fertility, what about the very fertile women who gets pregnant at the drop of a hat and needs contraception? I was one of these women. I tried the pill and it just made me sick. I tried condoms, and they just burned and hurt and took the pleasure out of sex. So I resorted to natural contraception and tried the rhythm method and conceived my second daughter while doing this. How could I have become pregnant on day six of my cycle, I wondered?

I was baffled for many years by this until I came across Francesca Naish's book called *Natural Fertility Management*, in which she recommends three methods all in one, to assist with contraception or, inversely, conception. Her work combines the rhythm method with the temperature method along with lunar phase cycle. What is all that you may ask?

To explain, a woman usually only conceives one day of each month of each cycle: this is when your egg is released for fertilisation. The trick is to know, which day? Taking your temperature allows you to know when you have ovulated. The temperature drops on ovulation day, then starts to climb the day after.

But what about this lunar phase method? This was something new to me back in the day. It turns out that a Russian doctor discovered a woman can ovulate twice in a month, and this can be worked out based on the phase of the moon, at the woman's birthdate and time. The history of this can be found in Francesca's book.

What that means is when you become a menstruating woman, if you were born on a new moon, then every new moon you could have a potential second ovulation. With our bodies being 70% water and the tides being caused by the pull of the moon, this can have a tremendous influence on our bodies. You can easily see when charting a woman's cycle if she has ovulated a second time, as there is a second temperature drop and a second lot of fertile mucus which only usually accompanies ovulation.

When I worked out my own personal lunar fertile times, it was during my period and that answered my question of how I could have conceived near the end of my menstrual bleed. I had two ovulations that month, one mid-cycle and one on about day five or six of my cycle. I have used this method of contraception successfully since for myself for approximately 30 years now, with no further babies.

https://www.amazon.co.uk/Natural-Fertility-Complete-Achieving-Conception/dp/1863510540 search here for a copy of her book.

I have included here my article written for my patients wanting to prepare for a pregnancy.

See RESOURCE 10: Preconception care

Endometriosis and Adenomyosis

There has been a lot of research regarding endometriosis and adenomyosis causing so much suffering in women, and over the many years, I have had much success and some failure when it comes to these ailments. I believe imbalance of hormones is a large factor, along with inflammation, toxicity, stressful lifestyles, and trauma having a lot to do with the causative factors here.

But there is another causative factor which is largely overlooked, with research being carried out by medical specialists in the field of gynaecology; that is medical procedures being the iatrogenic cause of these conditions, especially in the case of adenomyosis.

Any damage to the uterus lining has been scientifically established to be caused by laparoscopic surgeries, cesarean section surgeries, and D and C procedures, in which a metal instrument is used to scrape out the inside of the uterus, as opposed to the gloved hand. In doing so, there is enough damage to the uterus wall to cause adenomyosis to begin to develop.

As an example, one of my patients recently had a hysterectomy to end the severe pain and suffering she endured each cycle for years. This pain began after her cesarean sections. We tried everything for a few years: we balanced her hormones; made sure she was viral, bacterial and fungal free; made sure she was nutritionally balanced. She exercised regularly and had regular osteopathic work done on her lower back. She has had her children, now she is no longer in pain post-surgery. Thank you, surgeons!

To round out this section, I must take some time to mention some other methods of contraception such as the pill or implanon – the rod implanted into the arm of women which releases synthetic hormones to prevent conception by stopping ovulation, much the same as the pill does.

The pill puts a woman into an artificial state of pregnancy, with such side-effects as oestrogen dominance. This requires you take, month after month, year after year, high doses of synthetic hormones to stop pregnancy. Some women don't even stop the synthetic hormones to allow a bleed each cycle and feel that it is fine to go months without a period (or even years) and no importance is given to having a break from these synthetic hormones.

I have found the opposite to be true in my practice: it is vital to have a break and allow ovulation to occur at times. What are the consequences of altering the natural cycle without regard to the impact on a woman's body?

Not to mention – the opinion of myself and many natural practitioners being – *why not* use a more natural method of contraception with no side-effects or why not *address* the underlying cause of her hormone imbalance? Especially *if* that woman is taking the pill, to stop her period pain or premenstrual symptoms, which can be so severe. It is known as PMDD, Premenstrual Dysphoric Disorder and can cause both emotional and psychological distress to women each month before or during her menstrual cycle.

Some of the side-effects I have directly seen from use of the pill include overgrowth of Candida, a fungal yeast-type infection. This overgrowth can become chronic, leading to thrush, cystitis, constipation, diarrhoea, wind, bloating, nausea, sugar cravings, sinus congestion, increased hay fever, and even debilitating migraines.

The pill itself can lead to lower levels of vitamins B1, B12, B6, iron, and magnesium, to name a few. All too often this is combined with an increased emotional state, especially premenstrual depression, anxiety, acne, low sex drive, and worst of all, for a lot of women, weight gain.

For myself as a practitioner, I feel that the pill, like any hormone replacement therapy (HRT), can lead to an increased risk of hormone-fed cancers, especially breast, ovarian, and uterine cancers. These cancers are driven by hormones, and the high hormone build-up in the body can be a contributive factor in these types of cancers.

What I find most common in my practice is the women report their doctor does not warn them of any of these risks, even when there is a family history of these hormone sensitive cancers.

See references from the 'American Cancer Institute' and the famous 'Mayo Clinic' also confirming these risks.

This hormone imbalance can lead to infertility, repeated miscarriages, endometriosis, or cervical cell dysplasia (abnormal cells of the cervix). One opinion I have is the HRT (of which the pill being one) can lead to a further shutdown of the woman's body due to not *needing* to produce these hormones and so leads to a worsening of her PMS symptoms should she dare to come off the pill 10 or so years later.

Andropause, Perimenopause, Menopause

Andropause

Andropause, the male menopause, is a drop in the male hormones, and can start as early as 48, 49, or 50 years old, or does not occur until 60 years old in some men. These andropause symptoms are rarely spoken of, but the lowering of testosterone, androsterone, and/or DHEA can lead to greater visceral fat (belly fat), lower moods – grumpy old men syndrome – less tolerance of others, tiredness, insomnia, and even hot flushes along with depression. Men don't speak of these symptoms, but you would be surprised how many men are being prescribed antidepressants instead of getting advice and support for their male hormone reduction, even taking some medicines to boost their male hormones through these later years may be necessary.

I have also found such cases of impotence, the inability to hold or have an erection, lack of sex drive, increased inflammation – leading to arthritis and general aches and pains – are also very common problems in males suffering andropause. It is this lowering of these hormones in later life that can lead to a lot of these symptoms in men.

So what can be done about it?

Certain herbs can support and even assist in boosting testosterone, especially *Tribulus officinalis*, horny goat weed, damiana, and ginseng to name a few. I have witnessed success with evening primrose oil which is needed for the production of these hormones. Also, zinc, fish oils, B vitamins, and, of course, increased exercise assists in boosting hormones and is also great to combat depression.

Additionally, older men having someone to talk to and having support while they are going through these changes is important. It is just not spoken about enough, if at all.

One of my own patients was laughed at during work one day by a woman for saying how *he* understood what *she* was going through regarding her menopause. She scoffed at him saying, "How would you know? You're just a man!" Well, it turned out he had come to me with hot flushes, depression, tiredness, and low self-esteem. What we found in his case upon further investigation was low levels of male hormones. Just acknowledging that this was happening to him really lifted his spirits, and when he found out we could help him with this situation, he was just ecstatic. He, like many, men had no idea andropause was a real thing!

Perimenopause

Perimenopause can start as early as 41 or 42 years old for some women and go on for 10 years. Perimenopausal women can experience the beginnings of osteoporosis, known as osteopenia, due to the lowering of their progesterone, which seems to start dropping many years prior to their oestrogen, though, of course, there are always exceptions. From my observation, these hormones, especially progesterone, start to drop around 35 years old and manifests as such things as a lower sex drive or increased severity of premenstrual symptoms, such as heavy bleeding, clotting, and increased period pain, sore breasts, and headaches just before or just after the menstrual cycle. Sometimes the cycle is shortened or lengthened by several days, even missing a cycle completely.

Anxiety can also be a symptom and, in some, cause very low moods with tears flowing over nothing or everything. This crying is typically diagnosed as depression by the local GP, but instead of addressing their hormone imbalance, they are more often than not prescribed antidepressants and told they have depression or anxiety disorder or bipolar or premenstrual dysphoric disorder and sometimes told maybe they are just tired from raising their family and looking after the children.

The GP's solutions for many perimenopausal women is "take painkillers; take sleeping medications; go on a holiday – just use antidepressants as the solution – there are no side-effects and they aren't addictive." I know these statements to be given, as I have heard this time and time again from my female patients seeking real answers to what was happening to them. Also, if they are not prescribed these medications or perhaps anti-anxiety drugs, then most of the time they are told to go on the pill and just skip their period altogether.

This perimenopausal phase is a time that 'Metabolic Syndrome' can begin to set in, along with high blood pressure, greater risk of high cholesterol, and cardiovascular disease. Here is where the lower carb diet can be very useful and chromium to curb sugar cravings caused by the up and down insulin and blood sugar swings. Here I use mature hops extract of three organic bitter acids known as 'pHIX' that can reduce the belly fat, accompanying this metabolic slowdown that causes aging and reduction in our hormones. Also intermittent fasting can be of great assistance when it comes to metabolic syndrome.

How can you mess with a woman's cycle that much by using synthetic hormones to manipulate the woman's body and expect that body to have no side-effects?

So the question often asked by these women is *"which doctor* do I go to for help?"

Over the years, I have treated many such women and instead of blindly giving a one-cure-fits-all, I have listened to their issues and found the Naturopathic way to help them. My answer is, you need a Naturopath or a functional medicine practitioner to guide you through the more natural health solutions *first*, including wild yam creams, then perhaps bio-identical hormones next, and as a last resort, synthetic hormones if nothing else has helped to obtain relief and stability of moods during the cycle.

Menopause

Menopause can occur at any time from 48 to 55 years old for a lot of women, and I have an abundance of both knowledge and experience in this area as I am 65 years old and I am still managing my own menopausal symptoms.

For me, it began with flu-like symptoms so strong I was convinced I was coming down with a bad virus, which I have only had once in my life. My body ached; I was unnaturally exhausted; I was hot and, in a sweat, almost constantly; I was running a fever; and I had a mild, constant headache. I was out with a girlfriend one night who asked me how I was doing. I said, "I don't know what's wrong with me. For days, I have felt like I'm getting the flu, but I haven't developed a head cold or cough or sore throat." She looked at me and asked, "Do you think it's your hormones? You know, menopause?" I looked at her in disbelief and said, "No way. This is way too severe."

But when I went home that night, exhausted, and I really thought about it. I then realised I was one week overdue for my period, and because I was always on time; I never experienced premenstrual symptoms, not even period pain. I had not been concerned about keeping track of my cycle except for contraception reasons. It never dawned on me that I would have a hard time with menopause!

So I went into my own clinic that night and got my natural progesterone cream, rubbed on ½ teaspoon into the soft skin areas, and the next day, I woke up with a period. Half of my symptoms were gone.

My goodness, my girlfriend was right! I thought to myself. Menopause can't be this bad, surely? At that moment I had complete compassion for all those women coming into my clinic sitting down and bursting into tears, telling me they just couldn't go on feeling this way. I had a whole new respect for these poor women and what they were suffering.

Of course, I had been helping them year after year, but there is nothing like experiencing something for yourself rather than just watching it, to *really* understand just how debilitating menopause can be for some women.

Suffice it to say, I went onto feeling pretty good again, so I stopped my herbs and creams. But within a few days, I was back feeling terrible again. I then realised this really was menopause.

At this stage, I was running two practices in Melbourne, a drug and alcohol rehab centre in the Yarra Valley, plus I was doing volunteer work: helping others at my church with consulting and counselling. I knew I had to be relentless in dealing with this if I wanted to keep working 70+ hours a week and cope with these symptoms.

Here is what I have found really works for menopause: extra moderate exercise, getting body fat content down, and being mindful of not eating concentrated sugars and cutting out processed carbs (especially white flour and, in particular, wheat) and not drinking much alcohol at all.

Herbal medicine is really important, especially Chinese herbs and such herbs as false unicorn, black cohosh, dong quai, kudzu root, *Ziziphus* (Chinese date), *Bleuplurium, Hypericum* (St John's Wort), vitamin E, and activated B Vitamins. These address anxiety and the lowering of oestrogen as well as the lowering progesterone, the insomnia, and importantly, strengthening the woman's nervous system to help her tiredness.

There are many wonderful herbs that help balance and encourage a woman's pituitary gland to function at its optimal level, and adrenals must take a front seat here. This is because when a woman's ovaries begin to decline in their hormone output, then so too her adrenals can, and these are supposed to take over some of that oestrogen function. If you have adrenal stress or adrenal fatigue, then you are going to have stronger hot flushes because the adrenal output is also too low.

DHEA is one of those adrenal hormones that is a precursor to making testosterone, progesterone, and oestrogen. If your DHEA output has dropped, as it can in later life – 50, 60, or 70 years old – then you are in for a more rapid aging process and at much higher risk of osteoporosis. This goes for males as well. Stress is another situation which reduces your DHEA, and in turn, this reduces your testosterone, with all those side-effects.

The longer a woman can menstruate, the less likely she is to develop osteoporosis and the less aged she looks as well. Eyesight is another part of the body affected by menopause. You would be shocked to find out how many women become dependent on glasses after menopause sets in or as they were going through the ending of their menstrual cycle we call perimenopause.

A mention here about thyroid because it seems it is not recognised enough. As a woman ages and goes through menopause, it is not only her ovaries that are affected but also her whole endocrine system, and especially her thyroid. When your thyroid starts to become underactive, you can experience night sweats, changes in body temperature, tiredness, weight gain, thinning hair or just excess hair loss, anxiety, heart palpitations, and digestive inflammation leading to wind or bloating. Lowered immune function is also common, and so suddenly a woman of a certain age is getting every little illness her grandchildren bring home.

This can all be attributed to menopause, the only direction taken by your GP is the *female* hormones. I personally like to see thyroid-stimulating hormone (TSH) blood test results close to 2.0 or below in the Australian measurement standards; then I know the thyroid is efficiently functioning. But if it is 4.2 and still within range, the GP and pathologist will most likely tell you that your thyroid function is normal and there is nothing wrong. Yet this may not be the case at all!

I take one look at a blood test from a functional pathology point of view and know there is a sluggish thyroid here that needs support with such things as iodine (which Australian soil is very low in) and vitamin D. We as practitioners know that 1000 IU of vitamin D per day is not enough if your thyroid is not efficiently operating. Especially in winter, I recommend at least 5000 IU per day, or more, when vitamin D is extremely low.

Plus, I love to use tyrosine, an amino acid that supports T3 and T4 production. These are the two thyroid hormones that assist the body in so many ways. It is your liver that is responsible for this conversion of T4 to active T3, so if we also have weight gain around the middle, this could mean that your fatty liver is involved with an underactive thyroid.

A fatty liver is often a side-effect of weight gain, and this infiltration of adipose tissue (fat) throughout your liver is impairing the liver's ability to function efficiently. This in turn compromises the liver function in regards to the conversion of T4 to active T3.

There is one more thyroid hormone our body makes called 'reverse T3'. If too high, it can also impair your active hormone T3 with the resultant weight gain, tiredness, impaired female hormone function, and night sweats.

This means treating both the liver and the thyroid can very much assist menopausal symptoms, along with overall health and wellbeing and the correction of your adrenal gland and balancing female hormones.

Remember, as we go into menopause it's not just our ovaries that are involved with this change of life but also our adrenals, pituitary, and thyroid function as well! So a visit to your well trained Naturopath or integrative GP can help you achieve a more wholistic approach to menopause.

See RESOURCE 11: Diet Post Menopause

See RESOURCE 12: Birth Plan

See RESOURCE 13: Weight Loss Plan

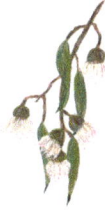

6

Cancer: A Foot in Both Camps

I could make this chapter the size of a whole book. I have treated, supported, experienced (personally within my own family), plus helped good friends and many of my patients with cancer to not only survive, but go on to live life to the fullest extent and for many years to come.

My 45 years of experience has shown me that when it comes to cancer, there is no one-answer-fits-all solution. The patients that I have seen that only do medical handlings alone often don't make it. Then there are patients I have seen who choose to exclusively apply natural medicine treatments only that also don't make it.

Then I have seen patients that only do medical treatment of drugs, surgery, and radiation that do make it, and then there are many stories of patients with cancer that used only natural medicine with radical dietary changes and lifestyle improvements – and they made it without any medical intervention. I have seen that too in my own practice.

So what *is* the best approach? Which doctor do you seek out when you are faced with cancer?

My answer is both…

Why risk just one modality when both have had success? Who is to say that your type of cancer will respond to either of the treatment protocols? It is often unknown how your body will or will not respond. You sometimes never know until you begin the actual treatment.

I have seen babies with cancer not responding to chemotherapy and I have seen babies undergo surgery and radiation only to see the cancer return. Conversely, I have seen those same cancers in babies and children – whose parents did both modalities despite the doctors giving them a very slim chance of survival – and those children went on to make a full recovery.

In my own family's case, we were given only a 30% chance of survival for my nine-month-old baby granddaughter, who then went on to experience a full recovery, flourishing, prospering, and leading a well and healthy life many, many years after treatment. In her case we used both natural and medical treatments concurrently. She has just turned 9 years old. My own mother used both modalities in her 50s and her bowel cancer was over 40 years ago. At 91, she is still cancer-free.

Whilst the cookie-cutter approach in allopathic medicine works for some, it definitely does not work in all cases. Often the patients that do make it are chronically fatigued and in some sort of pain for many, many years after their chemotherapy, radiation, and surgery is completed.

A patient's chances of survival with no return of cancer can be greatly increased with radical dietary changes and the inclusion of natural herbs, minerals, vitamins, and amino acids being supplemented either into feeding tubes or into smoothies while undergoing medical treatment and long after medical treatment has ceased.

Even the use of probiotics, the good bacteria in the gut, is important for the immune response of our bodies. We are hearing about the importance of our microbiome in immunity these days. Naturopaths have known this for a hundred years on more, with books written in the 1800s hundreds stating all health begins in the gut!

Firsthand, I have seen tremendous improvement in children and adults undergoing these medical procedures and treatments, with heavy doses of chemical medicine completely annihilating the mucus membranes of the whole digestive tract and suppressing the production of red and white blood cells, causing the loss of hair and greatly increasing the risk of secondary infections, doing so much better with the inclusion of probiotics, my granddaughter being one included here.

With the use of herbs and other supplements, their bodies noticeably handle chemotherapy, radiation, and surgery considerably better, bounce back much faster, so medical intervention can continue its work. Some integrative medical professionals have estimated a 60% increase in complete remission as a result of having a *foot in both camps*, along with far less risk of reoccurrence of their cancer in the years to follow.

I recently had a patient that had completed her breast cancer radiation. The nurses and doctors could not believe how good the skin on her breast looked and how well and fast she healed after each radiation session. Of course, she was on a lot of herbs and other supplements while applying ASEA gel and a silicone-based false skin onto her breast area, along with our *Skin Aid* ointment.

I have developed this ointment myself and have been prescribing it over the last five years.

The use of a silicone-based thin skin type covering over her breast while having radiation also really improved the outcome of the adverse effects of targeted radiation. All of her blood work was even in perfect range! The doctors were so happy but could not understand. Why or how did this happen?

Go here to source my skin Aid **https://naturalskinaid.com.au/** *and for info on ASEA gel go to www.asea.com*

The pine needle extract, 'Taiga', from a European pine tree, has been used in Russian hospitals for many, many years, in conjunction with chemotherapy and radiation, showing research statistics of a 40% to 60% improvement in the red and white blood cell counts of their patients compared to those same patient results without the use of Taiga also undergoing chemo or radiation.

Zinc and vitamin D have also been shown in vitro lab results to open up cancer cell receptors and increase the effectiveness of chemotherapy and radiation on application.

I used vitamin D, zinc, and amino acid protocols in the program for one of my own family members while they were undergoing a bone marrow transplant. Her outcome was a 100% acceptance of the donor stem cells with zero reaction in her body. Not only is this a good result, but her regrowth of these new stem cells in her bone marrow increased by

98% after only three months, which, of course, surprised the doctors, as it usually takes up to 12 months for this regrowth to occur in the majority of bone marrow transplant cases. This in turn meant her immune function and production of red and white blood cells were back to normal in very short order.

In the book *Radical Remission* by Kelly A Turner, PhD, she outlined 10 factors that were found to be common in all 17,000 radical remission cases interviewed. In this book, the cancer survivors, many of whom had suffered a reoccurrence of their cancer, had beaten it yet again, went into complete remission, and then went onto experience full lives with energy and purpose in life.

Once medical intervention and treatment has been completed, it is then the job of the patient and practitioner to detox and rebuild immunity for both prevention and restoration of their full vitality and energy.

Dietary changes

This is a very confusing subject for cancer patients in general, but the free radical damage (caused to healthy cells in their body), while undergoing surgery, chemotherapy, and radiation has to be dealt with if the body is going to cope with such aggressive intervention in cancer treatments of the medical models. It is not until it happens to you or a close loved one that you then realise that the medical treatment can be so harsh it may kill a patient.

See RESOURCE 14: Anti Cancer Foods

Like the series *100 years+ The Blue Zones*, on Netflix and SBS, showing the factors found around centenarian living to such an old age and all the while maintaining good health. They had no chronic disease, and their diets included high amounts of foods with antioxidants (whole foods), with no processed sugars or artificial colours, flavours, or preservatives. Their food showed lots of colour (greens, reds, and orange foods) and the majority ate a plant-based food diet with small amounts of meats. We often call this a Mediterranean diet.

Also, this approach can apply to a cancer patient: remove all chemicals from the diet along with high levels of sugar (which feeds the cancer cells and encourages metastasis-spreading of the cancer). Remove high salt levels, as some cancers have sodium as their metabolic pathway. Eat lots of organic fruits and vegetables with purified water. Good clean air to breathe is also essential.

I know the ketogenic diet (keto) can be of great assistance to fighting certain cancers but needs to be a modified keto diet because dairy products have growth hormones and are disastrous for cancer patients with tumours. The dairy products encourage tumour growth so the keto diet is managed by the Naturopath.

I would love to mention here a book on called *Earthing* or maybe you've also heard it as the practice of *Grounding*. This is getting your bare feet onto the grass, sand, or rocks and allowing the earth's ions to soak up into your body to reduce inflammation and pain. In *The Blue Zones* (also a book) there is a lot of description of people having their hands in the earth while gardening and exposing themselves to natural grounding.

Fasting is another approach to keep in mind and is only recommended with advice from a qualified practitioner. But certainly, a day before a chemo or radiation session, fasting can be great for reducing side-effects.

The key to beating cancer is largely reducing *inflammation* and boosting natural immunity while cutting out inflammatory foods like wheat, dairy, sugars, and too much red meats, which are high in histamine and can cause further inflammation. Cancer is an inflammatory disease. This is why exercise and swimming in the cold sea water and using herbs such as boswellia and curcumin in turmeric are also extremely helpful in beating cancer.

Next, I want to share with you some of the different modalities that can be incorporated into a patient's protocol to overcome cancer and be another one of the radical remission stories.

1. Herbal medicine, specifically the Harry Hoxsey formula, used in his 17 clinics around the USA in the 50s and 60s. These herbs were used by the Native American Indians when treating tumours. I will list my formula in the appendix.

2. Curcumin, propolis, boswellia, ginger, turkey tail mushroom, shitaki mushroom concentrate known as HACC. Curcumin (from turmeric) can be administered intravenously here in Australia by qualified medical personnel.

3. ASEA liquid, 60ml twice a day; ASEA gel topically and orally for mucositis.

4. Selenium, CoQ10; specifically, ubiquinol, iodine, vitamin A up to 60,000 IU, vitamin E up to 1000 IU, vitamin D up to 30,000 IU a day.

5. Vitamin C with bioflavonoid's orally up to 10,000 mg a day and intravenously vitamin C twice a week up to 40,000 – 60,000 units per infusion.

6. Hyperbaric oxygen for at least 20 hours, going up to 60 hours or more (120 hours for some). Can be daily or down to three times a week with hydrogen inhalation. Great while having radiation to reduce inflammation.

7. Light bed therapy, several sessions over a three-week period. This is where you drink a spirulina type liquid that attaches to cancer cells; then once you are lying under the light bed rays with the spirulina liquid, this targets and kills the cancer cells – the light being attracted to the spirulina attached to the cancer cells. This is both painless and has little to no side-effects.

8. Hyperthermia treatment, whole body or rectal for prostate cancers and rectal cancers. This is a medical procedure where the patient is under mild sedation and the body is heated up enough to kill cancer cells. Only to be done under medical supervision.

9. IV mistletoe infusions (again, under medical supervision only).

10. Stem cell therapy for repair of damaged organs after medical treatment and surgery is complete.

11. Parasite cleansing with black walnut, cloves, and wormwood (Artemisia) to name a few. This would also include ivermectin and fenben or menbendazol.

12. Juices, especially green juices and celery/carrot juice — always organic; you don't want to concentrate the pesticides.

13. Flax seed oil and digestive enzymes and probiotics for immune boosting and microbiome replacement/balance. Go to https://gerson.org/the-gerson-therapy for more info on this treatment protocol.

14. Enemas and coffee enemas. See the Gerson therapy protocols.

15. Cryotherapy can be added to reduce inflammation.

16. Hydrogen therapy, which has research showing reduction in tumours of the brain. Have a look at www.molecularhydrogeninstitute.org

17. Using sodium bicarbonate to make the body more alkaline. Some research is being done with direct injection of bicarb solution into solid tumours with promising results.

Of course, for each of the above modalities, I could write a long explanation about why they are effective. But it is good to do your own research. Ask your Naturopath, integrative GP, or integrative oncologist about any of these treatments that could be good for you and see what is available in your town, city, or area.

One of the fundamental principles in Naturopathy is having a low-acid diet and, of course, this is also a large reason why plant-based diets have been so successful for a century or more.

There is an acid/alkaline food list I give many of my patients. Staying on an 80% alkaline to 20% acid diet is one of the healthiest recommendations, not only for cancer patients but also for those with arthritis, autoimmune diseases, and digestive conditions such as colitis, irritable bowel syndrome, lactose, fructose, and gluten intolerances causing digestive issues.

Cancer cells do not survive well in an alkaline environment. It can become very technical to go into cancer cells and how they thrive, but for those of you who wish to understand more about the metabolic pathways there is a paper from the National Library of Medicine called 'Tumour PH and its Measurement'. Here we find information stating hypoxic cells (meaning low oxygen in cells) within tumours, as well as acidity produced just outside the tumour itself is the environment these aberrant cells thrive on.

This paper theorises that the high acidity production of tumours is likely due to the glucose metabolism of cancer cells in their growth and replication. This environment assists the survival of the cancer cell which is why hyperbaric oxygen can be very useful as an adjunct treatment for cancer.

It is forcing more oxygen intracellular in the body thereby reducing hypoxic cells and making it more unfavourable to cancer cells and their survival. This is also why ketogenic diets are receiving a lot of attention in medical fields. This diet severely restricts sugar and carbs which feed the cancer cells. But also hyperbaric oxygen reduces inflammation, which as stated above is what we are trying to rid the body of!

See RESOURCE 15: Acid Alkaline Foods

Pain

Recommendations for pain relief for patients with cancer can include; heat packs, infrared saunas, natural anti-inflammatories, as well as PEA (mentioned in the following chapter) that is for neuropathic pain/nerve pain. Curcumin from turmeric, as mentioned already, is a fantastic natural anti-inflammatory but can also be used for mitigating pain.

Hot and cold compresses are also amazing for temporary pain relief. Cold laser machine treatments, such as the one in my clinic, can be administered to the area of pain for relief. Acupuncture (either needles or laser acupuncture), can also be fantastic to reduce pain. CBD oil, the non-psychoactive part of cannabis, can be amazing for pain, stopping seizures, a risk in brain tumours, and for aiding sleep – so important in recovery.

See RESOURCE 16: Laser Therapy

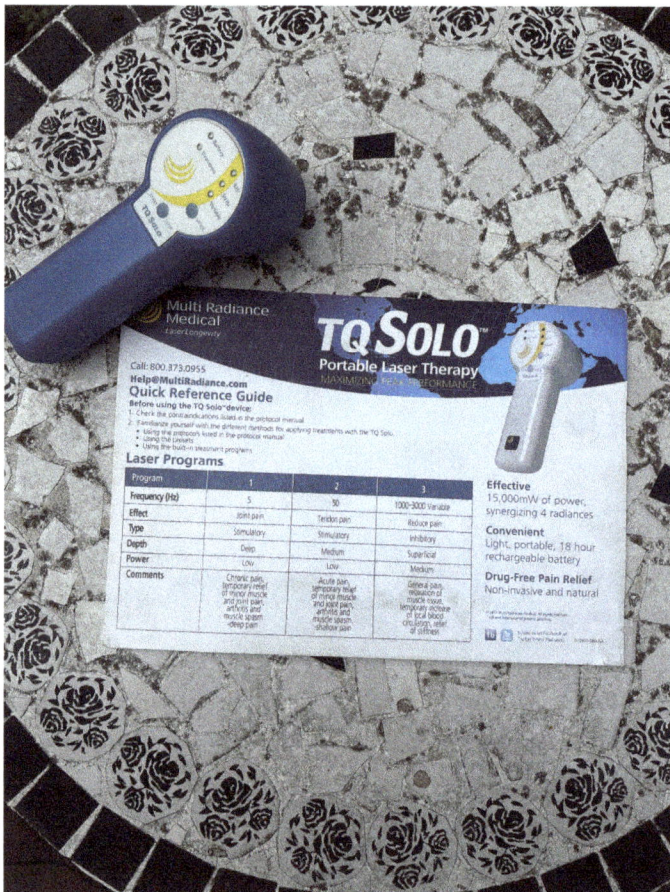

At times THCa (the more psychoactive part of marijuana) can be good for pain experienced with certain stages of cancers such as cancer of the liver, bone, brain, or sinus. This herb can be well tolerated often much better than morphine and codeine or oxycodone medications for pain. These medications can cause severe constipation, immune suppression, and even hallucinations and depression, all of which rarely happen with CBD oil or THCa oil given in such cases.

I cannot say enough about magnesium: it can calm nerve pain, reduce muscle spasms, and help aid a deeper sleep. Included for pain is an instant calcium magnesium formula made with boiling water to completely dissolve these two important minerals in a natural lemon citric acid base or apple cider vinegar base. Once these two minerals are in a solution, their absorption is pretty much instant and can act like a valium alternative to assist with sleep, pain, anxiety, and muscular spasms.

Melatonin can also be helpful if insomnia is an issue, and it is also known as being protective against breast cancer. High doses of melatonin are sometimes used in cancer treatments along with other modalities.

Now, it's all well and good for me writing about how to treat cancer using a variety of different methods, but we haven't really touched on how the patient may feel once that diagnosis comes back. Of course, a whole range of different emotions could manifest including anger, sadness, and loss. But all of those emotions are really just hiding the underlying fear: fear of cancer itself, fear of the medical treatment itself, fear of it coming back after you are given the all-clear or declared in remission.

Which Doctor?

So how do you combat this fear?

We all know that negative emotions weaken your immune system, so it becomes important to stay calm and find a sweet spot within yourself so you can sleep, not fall into a deep dark depression, and still be able to find a strong purpose to live – Not only for yourself, but for the ones who love you. It is important not to cry yourself to sleep every night thinking about the threatened loss and the ones you will leave behind and regretting all the things you did or did not do in your life.

Therefore, it is important you surround yourself with positive and naturally happy people and find what it is that will help you through these emotions. Be determined to stay calm and if that means having a professional to talk to, a best friend to offload to, or saying a prayer to bring you peace, then DO IT!

I have also observed there is a taboo surrounding giving patients with cancer, especially stage 3 or stage 4, hope. Is it because it is frowned upon, for giving hope in a hopeless situation? Are you are giving someone false hope or are you somehow deceiving them? I personally never believe the latter; it is hope that gives us the motivation and energy to continue on that journey and not give up but find strong reasons for living.

There seems to be an attitude out there somewhat like 'the pointing of the bone' in the aboriginal culture. Once the word **cancer** is mentioned, the big C, it is then expected that the worst will happen. This does *not have to be the case* at all and is not the case for thousands of patients.

I, on the other hand, have been very proactive in giving my patients hope because I have seen the worst cases survive against all odds, many times. There are a multitude of stories in so many cancer books of survival when all hope was lost. All those human stories of survival that we hear will inevitably bring many of us tears of joy and is nothing short of magic.

Who doesn't love a bit of magic in their lives? The human spirit is so resilient and can survive the most torturous pain and suffering yet live to tell the story.

So who am I to presume a patient will or will not live? I have long been disabused of that idea and the patients who love their oncologists the most are the ones that give them hope. Those who don't, shoot down their goal of beating their cancer. The doctor who supports what their patients have decided is right for them. So listening to your intuition if you are living with cancer and your own innate knowledge of what is right or wrong for you is also very important.

On a practical level, I tell patients there are non-invasive screening methods we can do every 6 to 12 months to make sure their immunity is staying strong and keeping an eye on their 'circulating tumour cells'.

CTC, as it is known, is a screening method which can be done with blood testing. This shows how many cancer cells you still have floating around in your bloodstream and can be indicative of increased risk of relapse or tumour progression.

Also, a less expensive blood test can be done called a lymphocyte cytology. This breaks down your lymphocytes to see the levels of tumour suppressor cells and B-lymphocytes and the level of your NK cells (natural killer cells). These natural killer cells are good to keep within a certain range to maintain a strong immune system. This gives patients a certain confidence they are doing well with less likelihood of any reoccurrence of their cancer.

I also believe having positive people around you is very important, so you are not having doubts seeded into your subconscious by the well-meaning glass-half-empty person that thinks it is better to prepare you to die than to live. These are the people that when you assure them that you're feeling great and even considering going back to work part-time, they look at you and question your confidence: "Are you *really* ready for that?" "Have you cleared this with your oncologist?"

You should distance yourself from these types of people. **You don't need them.**

I even recommend stopping watching the news, 99% of which is bad news covering death, destruction, and misfortune in the lives of others. This can be depressing for any person to watch day after day, let alone a patient undergoing cancer treatment. The constant flow of bad news and information can wear down one's resolve to stay positive and free from fear of your future, when one should be looking forward to your life and new adventures.

For some, it is having a positive, full-of-life best friend; for others, it may be going to church, counselling, surfing, walking in nature, mindfulness, a yoga or a Pilates class – whatever it is for you that is grounding and calming for your nerves, that which makes you happy, more peaceful, more loving, even joyful, then that is what you should do.

Oxymed Melbourne for hyperbaric plus NIIM Melbourne and go to oncolink.org for further info on hyperbaric O2.

Detox booklet available for those wanting help in this area. contact the clinic as required at naturalhealingcentre.com.au

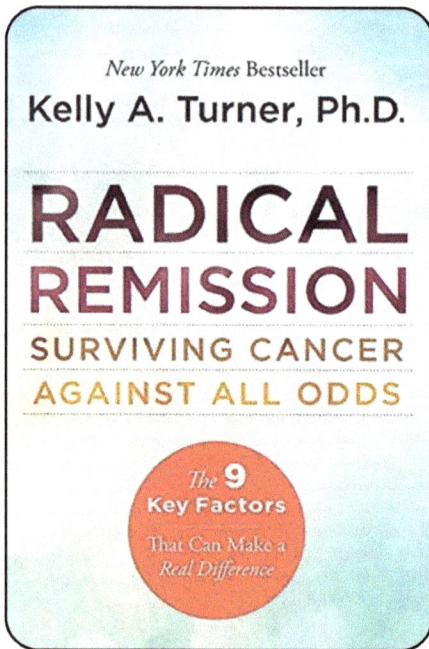

New York Times Bestseller

Kelly A. Turner, Ph.D.

RADICAL
REMISSION

SURVIVING CANCER
AGAINST ALL ODDS

The **9 Key Factors** *That Can Make a Real Difference*

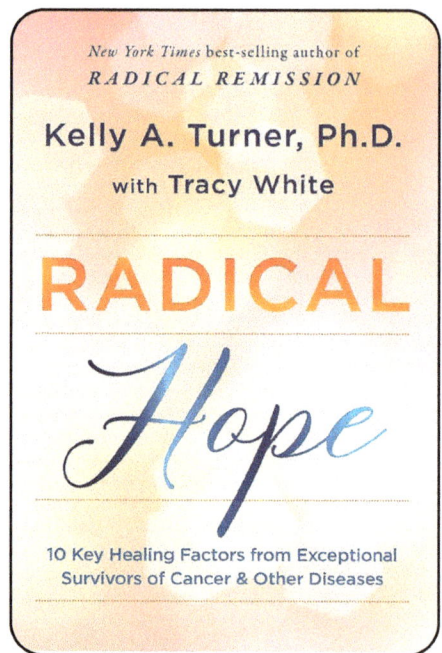

New York Times best-selling author of
RADICAL REMISSION

Kelly A. Turner, Ph.D.

with **Tracy White**

RADICAL
Hope

10 Key Healing Factors from Exceptional Survivors of Cancer & Other Diseases

See RESOURCE 17: The Cleansing Response

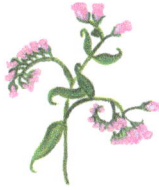

7

Anxiety, Depression, Insomnia – Alternatives to Medicating Yourself

I have spent a lifetime assisting patients with anxiety, depression, and insomnia. So many were completely convinced by medical professionals they must take psychiatric drugs or medical sedatives or sleeping medications, otherwise there was nothing else that could be done for them.

One of my patients described his experience of having been on strong doses of four different medications such as anti-anxiety, antipsychotic, and antidepressant drugs for over 10 years, as if he was in a mental straightjacket: completely numb. He said, "I was completely brainwashed into believing that I needed those drugs and that I had a mental illness and that nothing else could help. Now, I feel so much better being off all those meds and I can't believe what they did to me."

In this patient's case, he had also been self-medicating with marijuana and alcohol for his anxiety. This led to him feeling depressed and unable to sleep well, and in turn, this lack of sleep naturally only increased his anxiety. As a result, his GP and psychiatrist gave him antidepressants, which can (and did) worsen his insomnia, which then led to his depression worsening also.

Then, he was prescribed a heavy dose of sedatives to get him sleeping, which in turn worsened his depression. This resulted in yet another prescription of antipsychotic drugs as he was now being told he had bipolar and schizophrenia. This meant he was now being prescribed antipsychotic drugs on top of all the other antidepressants, sleeping sedatives, and anti-anxiety medications already prescribed.

He had kept drinking way too much alcohol in all these years, and by the time he came to me, he was crying during the whole consultation. He had not been able to work at all; his wife was there by his side nurturing him. Otherwise I believe he would have taken his life. This went on initially, appointment after appointment: the crying, the desperation, and pleading for help.

I just kept doing my usual protocols to balance his neurotransmitters and correct his nutritional deficiencies, all the while correcting his diet and making sure he had stopped drinking and smoking any recreational marijuana.

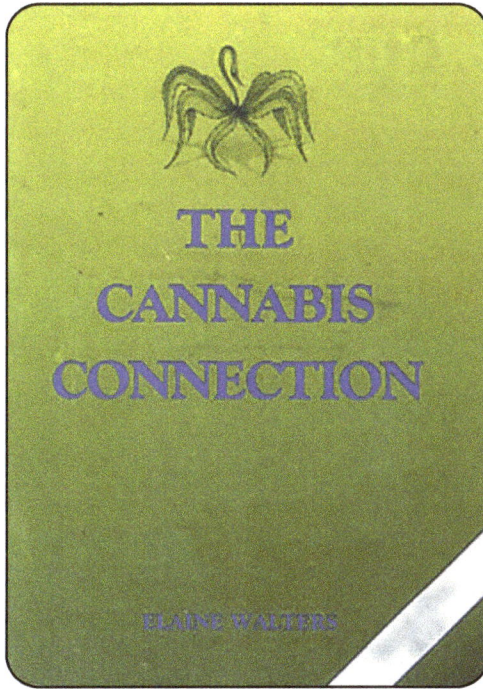

A good book outlining the risks and result of smoking a lot of marijuana.

At this stage, he was willing to do anything. So after I did an iridology analysis, I also checked his blood tests for liver, kidney, thyroid, and adrenal function. While he was with me during the consultation, I also took his blood pressure.

What I discovered was that he had debilitating back pain from the aftermath of a fall in which he had fractured his mid-thoracic spine some years prior. This pain was in fact the source of why he had been drinking and smoking dope so much: it was his effort to alleviate his physical pain and get better quality sleep.

So early on in his treatment, we did deep tissue massage and gently realigned his spine. I put him on magnesium and an instant calcium/magnesium drink plus a natural pain killer called PEA (Palmitoylethanolamide); a natural oil derivative from safflower lecithin, which is for nerve pain known as neuropathic pain, as well as being helpful in pain-induced depression. This medicine has also been shown in studies to assist the brain in decreasing inflammation. I also prescribed lots of high dose vitamin Bs, high dose vitamin D (as alcohol strips these from the body), and gave him extra vitamin B1 for emotional stability and his chronic grief.

We started food intolerance testing and desensitising on subsequent visits, and we found he had wheat and dairy intolerance, along with other food intolerances. These intolerances can and will exacerbate depression. I did gene testing only to discover he had MTHFR gene mutation, with double snips (meaning two genes, one from each parent, was mutated), resulting in his body NOT being able to break down synthetic folic acid, which is in most wheat-based products as an additive.

This gene mutation also meant his body struggled to metabolise toxins and to clear them from his system. Such instances of impaired methylation of drugs and chemicals like alcohol, caffeine, painkillers, as well as his psychological medications prescribed, meant he had a very toxic build-up and a lot of internal inflammation. This mutation also meant his body struggled to produce enough neurotransmitters. This alone explained his long-term anxiety as a young man drinking too much alcohol and marijuana.

See RESOURCE 18: MTHFR Gene Mutation

On top of this gene mutation, I also discovered he had high pyrroles, which are a by-product of red-blood-cell production and depletes both B6 and zinc from the body. We need these two nutrients to help make our serotonin (the relaxation and calming hormone), dopamine (the happy and motivation hormone), and melatonin (our sleep hormone). These together are neurotransmitters, or we can think of them as brain hormones.

These findings meant his body struggled to produce these neurotransmitters and even his male hormones. His very low serotonin and dopamine and severe adrenal exhaustion from the pain and alcohol abuse, along with the marijuana smoking, explained all his underlying causative factors leading to anxiety, depression, and insomnia and why he cried at every appointment.

See RESOURCE 19: Pyrrole Disorder

No doctor had ever researched the underlying factors leading to his anxiety, insomnia, and now, depression. In all his years of going to doctors, there had never been any offer of counselling by specialists or psychiatric doctors. Not once – which is shocking to think of, really.

This I see repeatedly in patients. He was not even offered any lifestyle coaching to assist him with exercise or sleep hygiene and there was no discussion of his diet and nutrition at all, not even questions about his alcohol or drug use. This patient felt wholly unworthy of his family, as he couldn't support them financially and hated that he could not work, which only compounded his mental health issues.

As the appointments continued, I went about helping him correct these neurotransmitter imbalances and nutritional deficiencies, all the while slowly, slowly withdrawing him off his psychiatric medications. He stopped all alcohol, marijuana, coffee, and painkillers and just used the prescribed natural medicines. We kept working on his back and his pain reduced considerably. He started to sleep much better and then started reporting, as his medical drugs reduced even further, that he was feeling clearer in the head, emotionally more stable, and finally, his terror-stomach, which he would awaken with every morning for years and years, was gone.

He had stopped crying at every appointment, and as time went on, he was able to go back to work part-time then full-time. His morale was up due to being able to support his children and his wife, who no longer had to be the sole breadwinner. The result of all this is, of course, is he is doing so, so much better. He still experiences a little anxiety, but we are continuing to assist him in getting his stress tolerance improved, managing his pyrroles and his gene mutation, along with his body's impaired methylation ability. He looked happier and so grateful for how much better life was for him and his family in those days following his treatments.

I tell this story because what I found in this case is not unlike what I find in many, many of my anxiety and depression patients. I find there has been no in-depth testing or real diagnosis of what's actually going on with the physical health of the person: no in-depth functional pathology work, no allergy testing, no food or environmental intolerance testing, no detailed lifestyle questions are being asked. No offer of drug and alcohol rehabilitation either! Experience has taught me that allergies or food intolerances will cause and can exacerbate depression as well as anxiety – A factor not well known or accepted.

I'll share yet another case in which one of my patients was anxious: he couldn't sleep; he felt tired and wired all at the same time. After taking down his history, I discovered that every day he was drinking 10 cups of coffee, drinking a litre of fizzy caffeinated soft drink, and smoking a pack of cigarettes a day – plus he was vomiting most mornings.

On his second visit to me, he came in singing my praises about how good I was and how much better he felt: he had stopped vomiting every morning and his sleep had improved a lot.

Well, you can imagine what I had prescribed: no soft drinks, cut down on cigarettes, reduce the coffee to two cups a day, start drinking purified water, and eating real food, not takeaway.

I gave him a probiotic for his gut, a multivitamin and… that was it. I honestly had to quietly laugh after he left because for me it was a no-brainer as to what was wrong with him. But like most of my other patients, he had been to the GP, and the GP could find nothing wrong with him.

If a person with a starving nervous system experiences these conditions of anxiety, depression, or insomnia, nourishing that person's nervous system should be the *first* priority, rather than sedating or artificially manipulating/altering the brain chemistry. Long-term sedatives such as benzodiazepines, antidepressants, sleeping tablets, or antipsychotic drugs should not be used as the sole solution to a patient in desperate need of help.

Of course, if there is a life-threatening emergency, then sedating or inducing sleep for a short time while investigation is underway by a wholistic doctor, Naturopath, or integrative psychiatrist is not only acceptable, but sometimes necessary. The trend for a long time now is this short-term emergency handling has become the long-term solution and I personally believe that is a lazy, unethical medical approach to mental health. These medical solutions, along with shock treatment and brain lobotomies, should never be conducted as a so-called cure. In my opinion, they are antiquated and barbaric methods of treatment for mental health.

Dr Mark Hyman in one of his podcasts was talking about sugar causing violence and mental illness. There are research studies showing the dramatic improvement in behaviour and even so-called mental illness just by cutting out sugar and processed carbohydrates. Anyone can search PubMed and find these research papers for yourself.

I feel that until all functional medical and natural diagnostic testing has been done and a causative factor or factors are found in each individual case, chemical medicine as a first choice is leading the population down a path of worsening mental health and a social decline. This is abundantly evident as the years and decades go by and the statistics show worsening levels of depression, anxiety, and mental illness overall.

According to the Australian Government statistics in their own website known as the 'Australian Institute for Health and Welfare', from 2020 to 2022, 8.5 million had experienced a mental illness at some time in their lives and 19% of Australians reported being diagnosed with depression, anxiety, or another serious mental illness in 2021, an increase from 11% reported in 2009. And in the younger population, the increase has been even worse from 26% diagnosed in 2007 to a whopping 39% in 2020 to 2022.

If governments took the money that they pour into mental health chemical-medicating programs and put it towards campaigns for eating healthy foods, cutting out sugar and processed foods, exercising more, and encouraging creativity, such as art, music, or sports, our communities would be a happier healthier and safer place to be in.

I feel so passionately against the ever-increasing medication of our society that I just must say something and do something to alert you. *If you are suffering, there are other ways and other means of helping yourself out of the depths of despair without numbing yourself, your body, and your emotions.*

As a patient said to me recently, "I have been emotionally castrated for so many years that I am having to get used to feeling emotions again, now I am off all my medications." This reminds me of the 2004 movie *Garden State*, where a young man is medicated by his father, who is a psychiatrist, from the age of nine years old, after having injured his mother and she ended up a paraplegic. It is the story of him coming off his psychiatric medications at 23 years old and rediscovering he can feel and experience emotions once again.

I call the antipsychotics drugs essentially chemical castration medications: the patient can't think let alone function at work or at home. They often feel nothing. They are living by default only, with experiencing an emptiness because they have largely been removed from 'present time' by the drugs they are taking. They may stop being a problem to their family or society as they become dumbed down and more vegetable-like, but they experience no real life. They are numb with nothing to look forward to, no goals, no purpose, and often no job, just relying on sickness benefits for the rest of their lives.

In a final note regarding depression, I want to mention something here about post-natal depression: why in God's name are the doctors not balancing women's hormones after birth? There is no real support there other than the prescribing of antidepressants. So why are they not testing hormones? Recommending counselling?

In my opinion, it is because they find it much easier and much faster to write a script for antidepressants than do any in-depth case history taking or testing to find the actual underlying cause of a mother's depression after birth. The general practitioner, too, has been sold by the drug companies that antidepressants are the be-all-and-end-all solution to their patients' complaints. The GP prescribes these drugs in the hope the patient won't feel the depression, but of course, she won't feel much of anything at all. So, I ask you, what happens to the possibility of enjoying the love, bonding, and getting to know a new life, her baby?

One of the alarming statistics coming out now is about mass school shootings around the world. Almost every single shooting is committed by people who are either on psychological medications or have just withdrawn off their medications.

The FDA further confirmed that antidepressants can cause violence in the FDA-approved Medication Guide for antidepressants. By law, Medication Guides must be based on science and on the drug's Full Prescribing Information. These several-page guides are intended to be shared and discussed by the doctor with patients and their families.

The FDA Medication Guide for antidepressants warns clinicians, patients, and families to be on the alert for the following:

- acting on dangerous impulses
- acting aggressively or violently

- feeling agitated, restless, angry, or irritable
- other unusual changes in behaviour or mood (Celexa 2017, p.33)

This list (above) of antidepressant adverse effects from the Medication Guide should make clear that antidepressants can cause violence. www.madinamerica.com

When I heard this, it did not surprise me. My experience of working with people for 20 years on antidepressants in my drug and alcohol rehabilitation centre is that they have little to no conscience. In other words, it is highly likely they feel no guilt after doing something they know is wrong. Reference can be found in the Citizens Commission for Human Rights website, the section in the film on antidepressants causing suicides.

Such atrocities are being committed all over the globe, and yet the drug companies that make these mental health drugs, and the psychiatrists prescribing them, are rarely being held accountable for these deaths and suicides.

So a word of warning to those thinking of going onto antidepressants: there are many other options prior to resorting to such heavy-chemical solutions as psychiatric medications.

Of course, counselling can be of tremendous benefit along with the more natural solutions.

A specific form of counselling has just been amazing for myself, some of my family members, and of course, many of my patients over the years. I think we all have baggage we carry from the past still affecting us in the present, baggage that is still holding us back from reaching our full potential.

To finish this chapter, I am going to list some of the natural medicines that can assist with anxiety, depression, and insomnia on a more physical level. Though please note, this is not an exhaustive list! While your integrative GP or Naturopath investigates the underlying causes of your condition, you can take this book along to your practitioner and ask about some of the following supplements.

SAMe (adenosylmethionine) 200 to 400mg per day is especially good for depression. This is an activated amino acid that assists the body to produce more neurotransmitters. Start using it every second day so as to not increase methylation detoxification too quickly if one is coming off chemical medicines.

St John's Wort (Hypericum perforatum) is a herbal medicine with studies showing that it can assist serotonin production and help sleep, as well as being good for nerve pain. This should be monitored along with your medication so as not to increase your serotonin too much and risk serotonin syndrome. I use this most often when a patient is almost completely off their antidepressant medication from the GP or psychiatrist.

Saffron, a powerful Indian spice, known to improve mood, reduce premenstrual symptoms, and improve sexual desire. I believe all this improvement is largely due to the increased micro-circulation to both brain and body alike. It can also assist with serotonin production.

Passion flower (Passiflora incarnata) is a herbal plant with substances that have a calming effect and can assist both anxiety and sleep.

Lemon balm (Melissa officinalis) assists in decreasing the stress hormone, cortisol, which helps greatly with anxiety and better sleep. It has a calming effect on your nervous system.

Ziziphus (Ziziphus jujuba or red date) is a Chinese herbal medicine that has been used for over 400 years. It can cause sleepiness and slow down the central nervous system, so it is great for the fight/flight response of the body in times of high stress. It also can be an anxiolytic (anti-anxiety) and natural painkiller. Unlike codeine or morphine, ziziphus helps the opening of the bowels and can be of assistance in constipation.

Magnolia (Magnolia grandiflora) is traditionally used in Chinese and Japanese herbal medicine for stagnation of Qi, the energy that flows through our bodies. It is used for depression, anxiety, and relieving stress while calming the mind.

Rhodiola is a herb which is great for the adrenals, both adrenal stress and adrenal fatigue, but can also boost serotonin which aids anxiety, sleep, and is known to assist with depression relief.

Kava kava is a wonderful herb for high-anxiety cases and very good for soothing the nervous system to aid sleep. I have used this in the most serious cases of anxiety where the patient was close to hospitalisation.

Calcium and magnesium, in the right form, has a muscle relaxant effect and can be a great alternative to valium for calming and relieving strong muscle spasms, which often accompany anxiety attacks. These attacks could possibly cause chest pain, headaches, or even migraines.

Patients often think they are having a heart attack, but when they go to the emergency ward, they are often told it is just an anxiety attack, and they ought to see a psychiatrist and go onto anti-anxiety medications.

Amino acids are also incredible for balancing dopamine and serotonin and producing more melatonin, your sleep-inducing hormone. L- Glutamine, taurine, phenylalanine to name a few.

While the herb *Withania (Ashwagandha)* can also assist melatonin production, your body needs B vitamins, magnesium, zinc, and SAMe to assist this neurotransmitter to be produced.

Melatonin is available over the counter and is a synthetic copy of our natural hormone. It is very safe to take when there is a deficiency of this brain hormone – I believe it is a lot safer than sleeping tablets or heavy sedatives such as benzodiazepines.

Very importantly, L-tryptophan and 5-HTP (the activated form) also assist in the making of these three important neurotransmitters.

There are rare times when a person has an excess of dopamine causing a euphoric state and ideas of grandeur. If it's too high, then the use of natural sedatives can help, along with alpha lipoic acid (a naturally occurring antioxidant rich in such foods such as tomatoes). Again glutamine, taurine and more importantly GABA (a neurotransmitter amino acid that down regulates and calms the excitatory pathways that keep us awake and in a euphoric type of state) is useful. I have found GABA great for sleep and anger in patients of all ages. It's best used at night.

Lastly, and somewhat most importantly, vitamin B. Deficiencies in B12, B-Complex vitamins, and vitamin B1 have all been linked to both anxiety and depression, as your body needs these vitamins to assist in the production of your own melatonin, the sleep hormone, that helps regulate our circadian (day/night) rhythms.

What is so amazing about using natural medicines is the body will use what it needs and excrete the by-products via your urine, especially when it comes to the vitamin B group. This is what makes your urine bright yellow when taking these supplements. If you feel that maybe it's a waste of money because it's just leaving your body anyway, it is supposed to be excreted, and it actually means it is being absorbed and it is helping your nervous system to be nourished and strengthened. Once ingested and used, it passes through your body in a matter of hours.

One must be knowledgeable in using the natural herbal remedies along with any chemical medications. But as long as you are not overdosing on serotonin and you are slowly stepping down off your prescribed psychiatric drugs, then there is no risk of serotonin syndrome. If serotonin is too high in your body, it can cause adverse side-effects. Be guided by your experienced doctor or practitioner when cutting down slowly on your chemical medication.

A note here on Parkinson's drugs: they too can be overprescribed by the specialists, causing too much artificial dopamine. So be mindful of using dopamine-boosting herbs along with levodopa, but usually, there is such severe dopamine loss in these patients there is little risk when using dopamine-boosting herbs and foods alongside of the levadopa medically prescribed drugs.

Such things as green tea, which contains L-theanine; a mood enhancer and chocolate-coco beans, can boost dopamine and can be of good help to the patients with shaking and stiffness that comes with low dopamine production in their bodies. Often, Parkinson's patients are depressed, so we as Naturopaths can assist these patients tremendously.

There is a good chart summarising the neurotransmitters, of which there are many more than the three I have focused on in this chapter, which I will add for your benefit here. Reference Dr Henry Osiecki founder of Orthoplex- Bioconcepts.

Serotonin	Melatonin	Histamine	Phenylethylamine	Endogenous Opioids
Functions	*Functions*	*Functions*	*Functions*	*Functions*
Control of eating/appetite Regulation of pain Mood Involved in regulation of arousal state and sensory perception May inhibit glutamate activity	Regulation of circadian rhythms Promotes sleep May regulate GABA receptor complex	Arousal and wakefulness Hydrochloric acid production Appetite, eating and drinking behaviour May modulate other neurotransmitters	Alertness Mental activity Inhibit breakdown of endogenous opiods Release or nor-epinephrine and dopamine	Release/modulation of dopamine, inhibit transmission of excitatory pathways Decrease pain sensation Reinforcement and reward Euphoria
Deficiency signs	*Deficiency signs*	*Deficiency signs*	*Deficiency signs*	*Deficiency signs*
Depression (worse in winter) Anxiety (incl's social) Aggression OCD tendencies Craves Carbohydrate Constipation (frequent) Low pain tolerance Poor dream recall Insomnia Impulsive tendencies Low self esteem	Insomnia Frequent migraines/headaches Fibromyalgia/Chronic pain Hypertension Tension/anxiety	Low stomach acid Food allergies Chemical/medicinal sensitivities Free floating anxiety Schizophrenia Depression Binge eating/drinking Fatigue/brain fog Low libido Social phobia	Depression Anxiety ADD Low pain tolerance Fatigue	Low pain tolerance Addictive tendencies Carbohydrate cravings Tension/anxiety Dwell over major life events Depression

Excess signs	Treatment	Cautions/Contraindications
Confusion Extreme agitation Muscle twitching Gastrointestinal distress or nausea	Individual nutritional and herbal supplements are available to assist in deficiency or excess conditions.	Antidepressants People with bipolar disorder CYP450 metabolised pharmaceuticals Benzodiazepines Anti-epileptic medications
May be due to cannabis use	Individual nutritional and herbal supplements are available to assist in deficiency or excess conditions.	SSRI's Bipolar disorder
Seasonal allergies Tolerant to pharmaceuticals Need very little sleep Schizophrenia Anxiety/Depression Chronic alcoholism Headaches Paranoia	Individual nutritional and herbal supplements are available to assist in deficiency or excess conditions.	Antihistamines Bipolar disorder
Insomnia Hypertension Migraine	Individual nutritional and herbal supplements are available to assist in deficiency or excess conditions.	PKU Antidepressants Benzodiazepines Anti-epileptic medications
Unlikely	Individual nutritional and herbal supplements are available to assist in deficiency or excess conditions.	PKU Antidepressants

Acetylcholine	Glutamate	GABA	Dopamine	Norepinephrine (Noradrenaline)	Adenosine
Functions	*Functions*	*Functions*	*Functions*	*Functions*	*Functions*
Parasympathetic nervous system Memory, learning, attention span REM sleep Release of gastric acid and digestive enzymes Peristalsis	Main excitatory neurotransmitter Memory Attention and concentration	Main inhibitory neurotransmitter Role in sleep maintenance	Motivation Mood Memory Movement	Arousal REM Sleep Concentration, memory formation Stimulates release or hormones that stimulate thymus gland May modulate firing of serotonergic and dopamine neurons	Falling asleep
Deficiency signs	*Deficiency signs*	*Deficiency signs*	*Deficiency signs*	*Deficiency signs*	*Deficiency signs*
Sympathetic dominance Short term memory problems Age related cognitive decline Constipation/digestive dysfunction Light sleeper & poor sleep initiation Holds tension in muscles	Unlikely	Anxiety/panic attacks Alcohol craving Seizures Insomnia Dwell over stressful situations	Addictive tendencies Tremors/restless legs Low libido Lack of motivation Depression Mental exhaustion Dull boring dream	Chronic stress/fatigue/pain Poor long term memory Depression Stress urinary incontinence	Sleep initiation

Excess signs	Unlikely	Agitation Poor memory, focus and concentration Mania	Unlikely	Aggression Schizophrenia	Panic disorder	Unlikely
Treatment	Individual nutritional and herbal supplements are available to assist in deficiency or excess conditions.	Individual nutritional and herbal supplements are available to assist in deficiency or excess conditions.	Individual nutritional and herbal supplements are available to assist in deficiency or excess conditions.	Individual nutritional and herbal supplements are available to assist in deficiency or excess conditions.	Individual nutritional and herbal supplements are available to assist in deficiency or excess conditions.	Individual nutritional and herbal supplements are available to assist in deficiency or excess conditions.
Cautions/ Contraindications	Anticoagulant medications Acetylcholinesterase inhibitors	Anticoagulant medications Not within 2 hours of antibiotics Renal failure	Barbiturates Benzodiazepines Alcohol	Antidepressants Lithium Thyroid disorders ACE inhibitors Diabetic medications Benzodiazepines Anti-epileptic medications Take 2 hours away from antibiotics	Antidepressants Lithium Thyroid disorders ACE inhibitors Diabetic medications	N/A

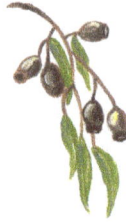

8

Allergies & The Immune System – Autoimmune Diseases

Where does one start with such an immense subject? It's difficult to know where to begin so as not to overwhelm you with too much information, all the while also giving you simple solutions that are achievable for most people.

In my practice, allergies and intolerances take up a large portion of what we as practitioners are faced with on a continual basis: from hay fever, to migraines brought on by foods, to environmental airborne particles, to chronic pain and inflammation in fibromyalgia, to rashes, chronic itching anywhere in the body, to gut reactions (IBS), to Crohn's disease, to ulcerative colitis, to asthma, to eczema – and the list goes on. More often than not, these are allergy-related conditions. Even diseases or physical ailments like neck pain, which are generally not thought of as allergy or intolerance-induced, when all factors considered and tests are done, the underlying cause found all too often is allergies or intolerances.

The first statement I wish to make on this subject is not well published or even understood. It is the fact that our immune systems have failed us, along with our adrenal/nervous systems when it comes to allergies.

They are the underlying cause for our allergies or intolerances developing in the very first place. These systems in a well and healthy individual will regulate our bodies when exposed to a food or a poison or an environmental toxin or any substance for that matter. Of course, there are exceptions such as the inherited intolerances from our parents or grandparents, but even these can be helped.

By regulation, I mean go into action to assist the body to deal with whatever it is. The nervous system gives the immune system signals to go into action and first attempt to neutralise the substance or toxin or poison by producing antibodies to block that substance's action. The white blood cells simultaneously go about attacking the substance in an effort to rid the body of the perceived poison, which is a similar response when exposed to a virus or bacterial infection.

The body then activates the adrenals producing cortisol and other adrenal hormones in an effort to reduce the inflammation that has occurred. The liver and kidneys, via red blood cells and the white blood cells, go about mopping up this explosive response in the body and will then excrete the by-products to bring the body back to homeostasis: the appropriate balance of the blood chemistry, the body temperature, and the heart rate.

Methylation is the process in which our bodies rid us of both metabolic waste and any toxins. It happens in the liver and is excreted via your bowels and kidneys/urine, even perspiration from your skin since these are our cleansing organs. When the body can't do this, the heart rate increases, the body temperature will first go up, and then the person can start to feel cold as blood rushes to the site of exposure. The person can then go into anaphylactic shock, but this will occur on a smaller scale even when you eat or drink something you are sensitive or intolerant to.

I know myself my heart rate increases whenever I drink alcohol. This is my body's response to the substance I have ingested. Parts of your body may swell up and this, in turn, can bring about an inability to breathe, as in the case of an anaphylactic reaction. Or you may experience an asthma attack or severe stomach cramps or chest pain as the muscles in the body spasm in response to the intolerance or allergy.

Hypoglycaemic reactions are also very common with allergic food reactions, which is a sudden drop in blood sugar after eating and can cause anxiety, shortness of breath, and a sudden feeling of weakness. All too often, it seems to me patients are being told by their local GP they are experiencing 'anxiety attacks' and then are prescribed benzodiazepines, a sedative-type drug, or anti-anxiety medication to manage what they are told is an anxiety disorder. Actually, in these cases, these patients are experiencing severe hypoglycaemia attacks.

These are but a few of the reactions seen from food or from environmental exposures.

In my opinion, allergic reactions are just named differently simply due to the severity of the reaction. If it is a mild reaction, we call it an intolerance. If it is more severe, we call it an allergic reaction. Finally, in the case of a life-threatening reaction, it is known as an anaphylactic reaction. However, these are all allergic reactions due to the body having had an adverse response to an exposure. They are all a protest by the body in varying degrees.

This begs the question: why? What is it that makes one person react, and yet another not so, to the very same substance?

The Naturopathic point of view narrows it down to your body's own immune system response, nervous system, and adrenal endocrine system not operating efficiently enough in order to help the body cope with the exposure. In a nutshell, your overall health and general vitality is compromised in some way.

Now, I want to make it known there are other factors that heavily influence a person's overall wellbeing in regard to allergies and intolerances, and these include the person's emotional spiritual state, their genetic-inherited health picture, and their nutritional balance. The latter may be caused by deficiencies often due to poor soil our foods are grown in – as well as the farming methods used to grow our crops, using lots of fertilisers, pesticides, and herbicides – and of course, our poor dietary choices.

All these factors, along with an accumulation of chemical toxins our bodies are exposed to, are called epigenetic influences, meaning they are influences on your body from the external environment. All these situations can influence the functioning of a person's immune, nervous, and adrenal systems, creating a perfect combination for ill health and allergies to develop.

I fully believe the first exposure of the body to such toxins comes from vaccines as a newborn baby. Substances such as polysorbate 80 (a stabiliser and emulsifier), benzoate (a preservative), or aluminium (a heavy metal nanoparticle used as an adjunctive and preservative), can initiate allergic manifestation. It is important to understand that nanoparticles can penetrate tissue and cells, therefore can go anywhere in the body. They are all injected straight into the bloodstream of our newborns right through until four years old, an example being the hepatitis B vaccine at birth. Even thimerosal (a mercury nanoparticle present in the flu vaccine), recommended each year for 4 years – then again at 12 years old – along with the introduction of boosters for whooping cough, hepatitis B, tetanus/diphtheria, repeated flu vaccines, gardasil for HPV and mRNA-type injections introduced in 2020, have bombarded the immune system repeatedly!

As a baby, I was given about 10 vaccines. The children of today are recommended to be given 52 vaccinations by the age of 4 years old – some of the same ones over and over again. *If you look up the National Immunisation Schedule (Childhood) you will see these recommendations there, just go to www. health.gov.au/childhoodimmunisation.*

Another source of toxins are pesticides and herbicides in foods and water. Even pollutants such as chlorine, fluoride, graphite oxide, and aluminium are in the water. The viruses we are exposed to, especially the latest viruses in our pandemic, leave us low in B12 and iron; this I have noticed in many of my patients.

We are also ingesting more food additives and food colours. Painkillers, anti-inflammatory medications, and artificial hormones such as contraceptive pills, rods, or creams contribute in succession. Furthermore, it's in our meats, chicken, and fish on sale that are raised in battery farms or farmed fish grown in nets that, again, are laced with antibiotics, artificial colours, and hormones forcing the growth to be faster, bigger, and fatter, making them more profitable at sale time.

Air pollution is also much worse as we breathe particulates from petroleum and diesel fuels…and the list goes on.

All the above can compromise a child or adult's health and wellbeing, including their immune response, which is why you may have noticed we see more peanut allergy and egg allergies in recent decades. We now have schools with a no-nut policy since the incidents of peanut allergy is so high in our children today. Why?

Did you know peanut oil and egg protein are part of the ingredients in some of our childhood vaccines? (I recommend you do your own research to verify the ingredients and additives in these childhood vaccines for yourself.)

Do you ever remember seeing or even hearing about peanut allergies when we were young at school, over 50 years ago? I certainly did not come across this phenomenon, so why now?

When a child has an antibody response to the vaccine, they can also have an antibody response to the substances the vaccines are cultured in, like egg protein and peanut oil etc… This is a reason as to why we have so many peanut and egg allergies in our children these days.

As stated earlier, we had around 10 vaccines at birth 60 years ago or so. I couldn't believe it was 52 when I counted them all in more recent years, but it is often the same vaccine, given up to five times during a child's first four years. Multiple different diseases are being vaccinated together in the one shot, for example MMR is measles, mumps, and rubella (German measles) all put into one dose, given now at least three times over. When I was young, they were all separate injections.

So what happened to the knowledge of trusting our own body's innate natural immunity to evolve and develop further and further in the first years of life?

Why aren't these vaccines being developed safer, cleaner, and without toxic metals included in them, which are well documented as neurotoxins and poisons to the brain and central nervous system? There is no reason why vaccine development can't be improved and the harsh chemicals in them removed. Go to *National Centre for Immunisation Research and surveillance* www.ncirs.org.au to do your own research on what is used in the childhood vaccines!

See also the Natural news article written on the influenza vaccine. Inside the leaflet, it admits the lack of study trials and the inclusion of thiomersal – mercury-based ingredients used as a preservative and the admittance of no safety trials done for pregnancy.

For what reason is there a blanket rule that all children must be vaxxed when we are all so different with very differing factors, as mentioned above?

Colds, coughs, flus, and other viruses; these illnesses are designed to strengthen our immunity into strong and robust systems to help protect us.

So the approach to dealing with severe allergy sufferers or even food and environmental intolerances is not a complex one.

For me, as a practitioner, it is simply to correct any deficiencies and give natural substances that will boost our immune systems while helping the person to improve their sleep, their food choices, the purity of the water they drink, their exercise regime, and to assist them in managing any stressful situations in their lives, all the while strengthening their adrenal response and nervous systems with such things as breath work, like the Buteyko breathing method, herbs, homeopathic medicines and nutraceuticals.

On top of this approach, I have a magic bullet to assist with immediate relief of an allergy or intolerance reaction, which I have already touched upon, known as Nambudripad's Allergy Elimination Technique (NAET).

Many years ago, because of promoting this fantastic technique on my website, I was fined $5000 by the Australian Competition & Consumer Commission (https://www.accc.gov.au/) (ACCC) and ordered to put up a red warning on my webpage for six months saying that my statement of assisting patients with their allergies was deceptive, false, and misleading.

This was despite the fact I had supplied evidence of such assistance to the ACCC, one kilo in weight of paperwork to be exact, showing improved bloods tests in patients after treatment, improved skin prick testing results, and improved lung function test results, all after NAET treatment. Ironically, the very commission that is supposed to protect the public from a monopoly told me there is no cure for allergies apart from cortisone and antihistamines – essentially, the medical model only.

The ACCC then enlisted 10 of their lawyers (all taxpayer funded), in a round table conference with myself and my one lawyer. When I asked whether they had reviewed, at all, the evidence I had submitted, which showed real help to patients with allergies in my practice, their response was – and I quote – "We have a room full of evidence to prove otherwise. Boxes of it."

They had not even bothered to read any of the evidence I had been asked by them to provide. They then continued with, quote "We have the head of the Australasian Society of Clinical Immunology and Allergy who is willing to testify in court that there is nothing else that can help patients with allergies" – unquote.

It was then obvious to me they had decided I was guilty before the mediation had even begun. They were not even willing to look at the evidence I had spent 30 hours collating and putting together for them, which clearly showed how treating patients using NAET was making a real difference to their lives.

I walked away from this mediation of ACCC lawyers and decided not to go to court to fight this attack on natural

9 September 2003

Nerida James Natural Healing Centre
431 Whitehorse Road
Mitcham
Victoria 3132

Dear Nerida

It has been some eighteen years since I developed serious breathing difficulties which necessitated hospitalisation, and subsequent retirement from work.

I eventually ended my hospital experience with a persistent productive cough, which was viewed by the medical profession as part of my illness. The little that was attempted to be done about the cough, was ineffective.

Over the years the cough led to painful muscle cramps, and increasing concerns of pulmonary and cardiac side effects.

It is now only four months since I first attended your Clinic, where I have received a combination of natural medicine and "NAET" treatments.

The cramps have ceased, I am less sensitive to the environment, and the cough has virtually disappeared. This has also enable me to reduce my traditional asthma medication. I have every reason to expect these improvements to continue.

With many thanks,

Light and Love

Roy Robson

medicine and the NAET technique, as I realised there was a very fixed idea. I also deduced since a medical-only point of view was being taken, I would not get a fair trial. After negotiating a potential $20,000 fine down to $5,000, I then had to agree to send letters out to every patient I had treated for allergies using NAET over the years, stating the practice of NAET was deceptive, false, and misleading, which was hundreds and hundreds of patients. Interestingly enough, not one patient asked for their money back and we received

189

phone calls and letters of support saying they knew NAET had helped them and how ridiculous this situation was!

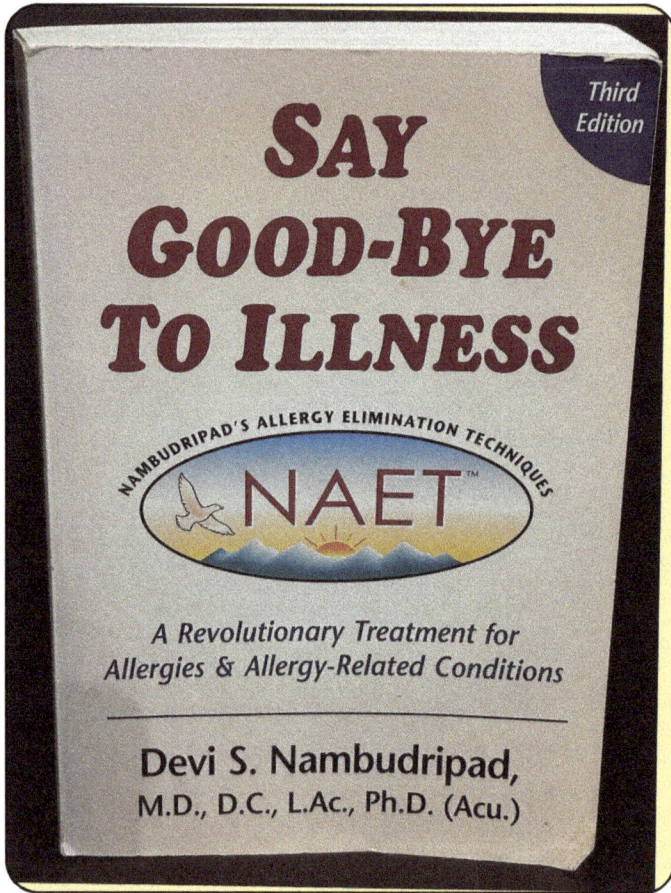

Of course, there are incidents when cortisone and medical antihistamines are life-saving, and I don't wish to take away from this approach at all; it has been life-saving for those patients with chronic skin conditions, asthma, and anaphylactic reactions causing near life-threatening situations.

My wish is for us to work together as there are times when the natural approach can say goodbye to illness completely rather than just managing the allergy situation for life. There are cases where the medical model fails completely, and it is only the natural approach that gives relief to a patient.

Autoimmune disease can be a devastating condition for a person to find themselves in.

Natural Healing Centre
8 Mt Erin Rd
Ferny Creek
Vic 3786
14/11/09

Dear Nerida

I am writing this to thank you for the incredible improvement in my quality of life.

When I met you in 2002 I could not hold a conversation because of an asthma cough despite being on three types of medication. I could not walk up my own driveway without becoming breathless and in need of a puff of Ventolin.

After determining my allergies you treated me with NAET and I have never been so well. The treatment removed my allergies which mean I no longer suffer from asthma. I take no drugs, eat what I like and now run up my driveway. In fact I now complete 'fun runs' of 5 – 15 kms.

The freedom to run without the restrictions of asthma is an amazing feeling and I know that NAET is responsible for changing my life.

A thank you is totally inadequate to tell you how I feel towards you and your staff.

But, thank you to you all

Please feel free to use this letter in any way you feel appropiate

Jan Bloomfield

The medical approach is to use immunosuppressant drug therapy, which I have seen to be a very helpful approach. But those patients are well aware of the potentially devastating side-effects of long-term immune suppression, yet never have I seen a specialist look for any underlying cause in these cases.

Like all disease, of course, autoimmune disease has a trigger, a set of physical or emotional circumstances that set off the body's immune response to attack a healthy organ or body part.

But I don't believe it can just come from nothing, so we should be asking ourselves, why? Why is it, for example, that a 14-year-old child's immune system suddenly starts attacking their pancreas and causing type 1 diabetes? I saw three cases of this not so long ago, and on investigation, I found it had occurred within months after receiving the vaccine given for human papillomavirus (HPV), Gardasil.

It is in my opinion that the immune response to this vaccine became exaggerated in that child's body and so out of control that the vaccine ingredients caused the body to attack *itself*, not just create antibodies against the human papillomavirus.

I've also seen this with viruses causing autoimmune response in patients, such as glandular fever (EBV) causing chronic fatigue syndrome and fibromyalgia post-infection. I've seen colitis and Crohn's disease manifest after gastro infections and parasite infestations, as well as after trips to other countries, where the patient became very ill and was suffering from severe diarrhoea for days.

There is a whole book dedicated to EBV causing Hashimoto's disease which is the autoimmune disease attacking the thyroid gland: *Thyroid Healing* by Anthony Williams.

He asks the question, "is this an autoimmune disease in these cases, or is it the body attacking a virus lodged in the tissues of that part of the body?" Or could it be from a parasite, or infection, which has the appearance, of an autoimmune response, I ask you?

I've done cleansing with these types of cases and administered antiviral and anti-parasitic herbs, in addition to antibacterial approaches, all to assist these autoimmune responses, in a concerted effort to calm the body's immune response down.

A good example of this is rheumatoid arthritis, which attacks the joints. There is a school of thought and research amongst medical doctors giving long-term low-dose antibiotics in such cases with promising results. But why? What is the antibiotic killing that is calming down the patient's immunity?

Leaky gut, known medically as gut dysbiosis, has also been traced back to being a causative factor in autoimmune disease. Using such things as bone broth and herbs to repair the gut wall and certain probiotics to assist in the control of the immune system response has proven successful in many cases.

All too often, I find food allergies or intolerances are a mitigating factor, and addressing these, while treating with other means, is also vital for the resolution of an autoimmune disease, in my experience.

I will sometimes do a gut microbiome mapping test, which checks for about 200 factors in your gut health and shows if there is an overgrowth of bad bacteria and/or a deficiency in good bacteria. It also reports any parasite overgrowth or infection from stealth pathogens. This is what we call functional pathology testing, and we are looking at the efficiency of the patient's body's function and operation, not necessarily disease. In other words, we are looking for an underlying causative factor.

This approach can often find that cause and extrapolate as to why that person's immunity has become out of control or overactive.

Do we really think the body was designed to attack itself? Of course not! There has to be a reason. And if we can treat that and cleanse a person's body of toxins, all the while reducing inflammation, by approaching autoimmunity in this way, we can bring about an incredible improvement in patients with these conditions.

See RESOURCE 20: Biogenetic Hair analysis

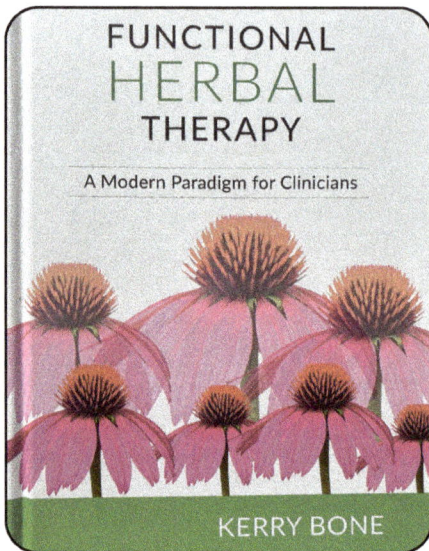

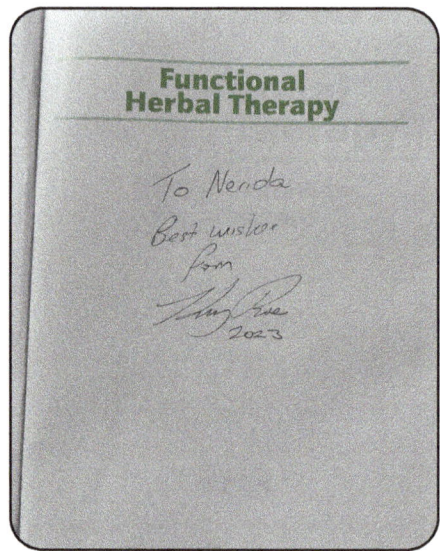

Emerald naturopath wins right to be called doctor

By Steve Theodore

Emerald-based naturopath Nerida Kalab scored a victory for her profession last week when a Frankston magistrate dismissed a complaint made against her by the Victorian Medical Practitioners Board (MPB).

Ms Kalab's dispute with the MPB arose in November 1993, when a Malvern medical doctor picked up a flyer that Ms Kalab had distributed to promote one of her clinics in Chelsea.

The flyer consisted a picture of Ms Kalab with the title "Dr Nerida Kalab N.D." written above it, and "Naturopathic Physician" written underneath it.

The medical doctor lodged a complaint with the MPB, believing that it was illegal for Ms Kalab to use the title 'doctor'. The MPB then passed the matter to the Victorian Criminal Investigation Bureau (CIB).

In April last year the CIB raided Ms Kalab's Chelsea clinic, at which

she was not present at the time, and interviewed a young female member of staff for more than 90 minutes.

Some months later, Ms Kalab received a summons to appear in the Frankston Magistrates Court.

But on Thursday last week, Magistrate Robert Tuppen dismissed the charges against Ms Kalab.

Mr Tuppen said that Ms Kalab was technically in breach of the old Medical Practitioners Act, which was in place at the time of the incident, but he commented that "so was his vet".

Mr Tuppen also said that Ms Kalab had an "honest and reasonable belief" that she was entitled to refer to herself as a doctor, because her qualifications include a bachelor of naturopathy after four years training at Laws College of Naturopathy in Ringwood. Ms Kalab was

also awarded legal costs.

"In July last year a new version of the Medical Practitioners Act was put in place, and the prosecutor actually told me himself that I wouldn't have been charged under the new legislation," said Ms Kalab.

"I feel it was a fantastic result, because the whole thing was so unjust - it was the vindictiveness of this one particular doctor who started the whole thing.

"A large proportion of the medical profession are very antagonistic towards naturopaths, and I think that's indicative of a certain insecurity on their part.

"I am only helping the public as much as I can, using preventative medicines, and I believe there will always be a place for both the medical and naturopathic professions."

Under section 62 of the current Medical Practitioners Act, it is illegal for non-medical practitioners to refer to themselves as a medical practitioner or medical doctor.

Emerald naturopath Nerida Kalab scored a victory for her profession last week.

AGE NEWS 17/3/95.

Naturopath wins right to call herself a doctor

By STEVE DOW, medical reporter

A naturopath has won the right to call herself a doctor after a magistrate dismissed a complaint by the Medical Practitioners Board.

Ms Nerida Kalaba, who calls herself a naturopathic physician and homoeopath and runs a clinic in Chelsea, was charged by police last year after a complaint was made to the board.

The board alleged that under section 28 of the Medical Practitioners Act, which was repealed last year, Ms Kalaba was not entitled to advertise herself as a doctor, because this could mislead the public that she was a medical practitioner.

But Ms Kalaba said her advertising made it clear that she was a naturopathic doctor, and not a medical doctor.

Magistrate Mr Robert Tuppen, in Frankston Magistrates' Court, yesterday dismissed the charge, finding that Ms Ka-

laba had an "honest and reasonable belief" that she was entitled to refer to herself as a "doctor".

This was because of her qualifications, which include a bachelor of naturopathy after four years' training at Laws College of Naturopathy in Ringwood.

Ms Kalaba said yesterday her victory was one for natural therapists. "The Australian Medical Association has tried to have a monopoly over health care," she said. "I see this as a win for the professionalism of natural therapies."

But Ms Kalaba's barrister, Mr Max Perry, said the finding may have limited legal application because it was based on Ms Kalaba's belief that she was entitled to call herself a doctor.

Under section 62 of the new Medical Practices Act, which last year replaced the previous legislation, it remains illegal for non-medical practitioners to refer to themselves as a medical practitioner or medical doctor.

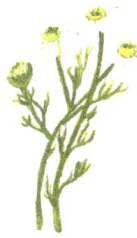

9
Energy Medicine: It Takes All Kinds

Now that I have been in practice for 45 years, I look back on all the modalities of healing and realise so many involve the manipulation of energy in order to heal the body or assist the body to heal itself.

For example, acupuncture involves needles inserted into the meridians: the 12 main energy pathways the Chinese discovered centuries ago that run through the body. By inserting these fine needles, it frees up the blocked energy in that part of the body, allowing it to heal itself.

In homeopathy, the homeopath captures the energy of a plant or poison or substance and gives it to a patient in minute, greatly attenuated, tiny, tiny doses. It is really capturing the energy essence of that substance, then giving small doses to influence the function of the body. The philosophy is 'like attracts like', so if a large dose of something causes that symptom in a healthy subject, then a minute dose will bring about a resolution of that same symptom in a sick or diseased individual. Again, it is taking something orally to affect a change largely through energy to heal.

Bowen therapy, too, is a flicking of the muscle to send a message through the fascia that lines the muscles, literally sending an energy message to that area of the body telling it to relax and realign into its optimal state.

Water therapy of different kinds also sends messages to assist the body to function more efficiently through drinking more water, to fasting with water only, to heat packs using hot water, ice packs using cold water to reduce inflammation, ice baths to reduce inflammation, and compresses to draw out toxins, such as in an abscess or splinter.

NAET, Nambudripad's Allergy Elimination Treatment, uses a combination of acupressure and homeopathic vials containing different substances a patient may be intolerant or allergic to. By tapping the acupuncture points down the spine while holding the allergen, we are affecting changes to the energy of the body and reprogramming the brain and immune system to understand that these substances are not harmful to the body and so to not overreact when the body is in contact with that substance in the future. This changes the energy through the nervous system, creating a more positive response in that patient's body.

I have used this NAET technique to help a patient to have medical insulin. Their body was no longer responding well to it, leading to other issues with certain foods, such as eggs or fruits that the patient could no longer eat. NAET changes the energy and improves the patient's circulation and immune response, bringing about a healing.

Chiropractic and osteopathy are in themselves techniques to free up blood, lymph and nerve flows in the body, so it can reduce inflammation and assist the body to heal itself.

Go here for more info on introduction to chiropractic videos. Https:// chiroshub.com/videos/

Laser therapy is something I use in my clinic that reduces pain and assists the healing of tennis elbows, bursitis of joints, and areas of arthritis. Laser is a type of frequency stimulating healing and encourages resolution of inflammation within your body tissues and cells. This too is energy.

Energy Medicine is a modality that is largely unknown. It is the ability of a person, the healer, to generate energy, much like what I discovered as a young massage therapist when working for the chiropractor all those years ago. The operator or practitioner just sits quietly, focuses and generates energy themselves, then focuses that energy onto a patient who is suffering, and puts that healing energy into that person's body in the area of pain or disease.

One of my patients had numbness in a part of his body, and after five minutes of energy medicine, he regained full feeling back in his body part, and this remained corrected weeks and weeks later. Another example is my own bookkeeper. She had ruptured her discs in her lower back, lumbar area, many years ago, and whilst she had largely recovered, she always had some pain and stiffness ever since. After receiving two five-minute energy medicine sessions from myself, her pain and stiffness have been 95% better, all after 15 years of suffering. She can now exercise much more without the fear of injury and has reported her lower back and abdomen are strengthening.

Energy Medicine is not some weird modality of bringing in spirit guides or God or waving your arms around or voicing incantations of some strange spell. It is *nothing* like that. It is having the patient or person you wish to help sit or rest quietly and relax while the healer focuses on putting their attention into the area where they have body pain or a condition or illness, then checking in with the person after a few minutes to see if what you have done as the practitioner is making a difference. We make no promises, and I can't help everyone, but I have noticed if I do just five minutes of the energy medicine before I realign the patient's spine, it is always much more relaxed.

The most famous healer doing this is a Melbourne man named Charlie Goldsmith who has had documentaries made about his work called *The Healer*, and he has produced some miraculous results, such as an 11-year-old with juvenile arthritis, whose pain was gone after one or two sessions. While he does one-on-one person healings, he creates amazing results healing from afar via Zoom, Facebook, or over the phone. He also does online Eventbrite healing sessions where he chooses three to five people from the 700 or more that are tuned in, and affects a healing on them via a Zoom link.

Charlie is currently in Los Angeles, USA, doing a trial within a medical facility with his results being documented in the hope Charlie can have this modality of healing much more accepted and known. It definitely is on the way to becoming more accepted as yet another modality of natural medicine to be employed when other treatments fail to assist.

I myself have started to develop my own skill in this area and see it as just another tool we as practitioners may use to heal where other modalities, such as allopathic medical drugs or surgery, have failed to help such diseases. These include autoimmune diseases, muscular dystrophy, multiple sclerosis and ALS: a disease affecting the nervous system, brain, and spinal cord, causing loss of motor controls. Although this motor neurone disease is being diagnosed as terminal, perhaps energy medicine can slow down or even halt the inevitability of this disease. I believe the research Charlie is doing in the States is vital in improving both knowledge of health and healing for our future generations. It is a truly remarkable and powerful tool with no adverse side-effects.

www.CharlieGoldsmith.com.au

I myself will continue to develop this skill to add to my extensive range of techniques used to treat the cause of disease. To date, I have personally treated about 80 people with my own energy medicine, and so far, there has been improvement in approximately 80% of these patients. For some, a miracle has occurred; for others, they have enjoyed a definite stable improvement to their long-standing chronic condition which has resulted in some form of debilitating pain.

Here is a text I received just yesterday about a patient. This patient has been suffering this pain for 10 years or more, along with bleeding from her bowel since her surgery and radiation. This is from her son. She is 85 years old and living here in Melbourne, Australia.

As you know, my mother has been suffering from heavy pain in the anus area when she goes to the toilet due to radiation damage to her bowel after colon cancer. She told you that the pain from 1 to 10 is usually about 8. Well, I asked her yesterday, how was the pain and she said it was a 2. This morning, I asked her again and she said it was a zero. So, so far, we are experiencing a miracle. Hopefully it stays this way. Thank you!

Another one of my patients injured her lower back 15 years ago and herniated her disc. At that time, I helped her to heal and got her walking with minimal pain. It had not been debilitating for her, but she always feels she needs to be careful, or it will seize up on her and cause her severe pain. Perhaps two or three times a year, she comes in to have massage and an adjustment much like servicing our cars to keep her on track. I asked her one day if she would like me to try my energy medicine on her lower back as she frequently has low-grade pain and stiffness, especially when working long hours on her feet.

She agreed, and as soon as I started, she could feel the energy in her body in her lower back area pulsating and moving around as I closed my eyes and focused there in her body. Her pain level was about a 5 out of 10 that day. Within three minutes, I had taken her pain level down to a zero. I said to her it can have a natural pain-killing effect, but we won't know for several days as to how much better she will feel.

I saw her two weeks later and asked how she was feeling in her lower back. She reported that the pain had not come back to a 5 but was sometimes a 2. She said she felt able to stretch her back more with no discomfort and felt her back strengthening as the days went by. So I did about another five minutes of energy medicine on her that day and checked back with her three weeks later. At this appointment, she said her back pain had completely gone and she was able to exercise more and stand much longer with no back pain at all! She said she felt like it had completely healed.

A more recent case came to me because she was suffering from a chronic cough that had been lingering for six weeks. Whilst she could feel it was almost gone, she still had a sore, irritated throat that kept flaring up and coming and going and she could feel it in her glands. She was taking all the right vitamins, herbal medicine, and minerals, looking after her diet – but still could not kick this throat symptom.

I did literally three minutes of energy medicine on her throat, and her discomfort and irritation was completely gone. So again, my advice was to let me know how she felt afterwards, and if it came back, she could reach out and we could work on it again. So far, it has been a month and there has been no sign of her symptoms returning.

Another case was a man who had two numb fingers on his right hand on and off for 10 years with his index finger, but his middle finger was completely numb for all those years. Five minutes of energy medicine and the index finger had full feeling and in the middle finger, 95% feeling had returned. Again, I made no promises but he was amazed he could feel his fingers again in such a short space of time.

He has checked in with me again to let me know after five days his fingers are still great and have feeling in them. I'm so happy for him. He has since now, two months later, checked in with me and his fingers are both fantastic. He was booked in for surgery, but it is no longer required. I have story after story of symptoms completely disappearing in a very short space of time with this type of healing.

At times patients do have the symptoms return but with 50% less pain, indicating further sessions are needed to get a good result. And sometimes, the energy medicine has zero effect, but the fantastic thing is? It does no harm, nor does it have any side-effects. It is very quick to work or not work, so you don't have to spend hours and hours before you know the outcome.

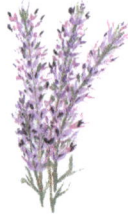

10

Stand-Out Success Stories

Awholistic approach to health and wellbeing is, in my opinion, the use of a combination of medical treatments, drug therapies, natural modalities, and natural medicines. These are all the essentials for the future of our health. To achieve a high success rate amongst a population that is marred with a multitude of illnesses and or diseases afflicting so many of us in modern society today, we need to be able to have more education out in the public domain so a person can decide which doctor they may need. It's also essential to have all doctors willing to refer to other modes of treatment if what they are doing is not working. Referral and having no reluctance or fear of referring is vital in achieving this goal.

Surgery for gallbladder removal in a patient full of stones, which is causing severe pain for that poor patient, is a godsend and so needed. The spiral fracture or compounded fracture of a smashed bone is nothing short of miraculous when the orthopaedic specialist works their skills. My hat goes off to these practitioners that dedicate their life to helping those in need.

But in saying that, there are times where these sorts of doctors or your local GP just can't help you with your migraines, your back pain, your infertility, your chronic fatigue syndrome, or your weakened immunity. The list goes on for people suffering who have sought the help of many a medical professional only to be told "You will have to learn to live with it," or "It's all in your mind," or "There is nothing more we can do for you."

How depressing must this be to the person suffering and being given no hope?

My advice is **never stop searching**. If one practitioner and one modality does not help you, perhaps another practitioner or another modality will help you.

It may be a simple **homeopathic medicine** or a **dietary change**, like **eat right for your blood type**, the **carnivore diet** or **ketogenic diet**, or just a single **herbal medicine** or a session of **energy healing** or **chiropractic** or **osteopathic** treatment, a **Bowen** therapy session or an **acupuncture** treatment. Maybe some **counselling** like **Dianetics**; perhaps **pilates** exercise or **hydrotherapy** water treatment exercises;

perhaps it's **myotherapy** (a type of deep tissue massage) and **dry needling**. Perhaps **Hydrogen therapy** (breathing this in with oxygen) or **EE System** (energy enhancement system of healing with bio waves/scalar waves). Perhaps **IV vitamins** (intravenous vitamin C, minerals, or antioxidants) or **laser** treatments for torn muscles, ligaments, or inflamed joints and pain relief.

My point being – there is no shortage of different approaches to resolving your issues and no shortage of practitioners out there. It is more that you have to wade your way through all the information so you can find your way to success.

I want to tell you about some of my successes over the years, just to give you hope if you need it and also to document just how much success one practitioner can see over many years in practice. This keeps me excited and passionate about my work and keeps me wanting to let the world know there is so much available out there to help you. Use your intuition, use your contacts: use your hope and determination to find what works for you. There are answers – they are out there; you just have to keep looking to find what is right for YOU!

About 20 years ago or more, a patient came to me after she discovered she had a brain tumour which caused her to have seizures anytime she had even a mild fever from a common cold or virus. After conducting some iridology and discovering her body was far too acidic (which was causing the severe inflammation in her brain) I put her on an alkaline-heavy diet: some herbs for tumour growth suppression, along with a lot of supplements for her brain nutrition such as magnesium, potassium, calcium (electrolytes), and vitamin Bs. Within six months, she had not experienced any further seizures, so she decided to undergo a second MRI brain scan only to discover her tumour was gone. The doctors were baffled and could not understand such a miracle. I am still in contact with that patient today: the tumour has never regrown, never returned, and she never had another seizure.

I had another patient that was diagnosed with uterine cancer which had been confirmed with biopsies, scans, and blood tests. She came to me for help prior to her scheduled surgery, and we did a cleansing for parasites and gut health. I also gave her detoxing herbs which have known anti-cancer properties and recommended a strict healthy-eating program. She went in for her hysterectomy and before surgery, they did another ultrasound to locate exactly where the tumour was only to discover it had *gone*! As a result, they cancelled her surgery that day, very baffled. One doctor even suggested to her that the original diagnosis must have been wrong.

Many times, I have assisted infertility cases only to have them conceive, even after eight years or longer of trying.

One of my beautiful infertility patients, whom I later taught natural contraception methods, went on to have four children. Another patient was told at a young age she would never have children by her gynaecologist. She was 19 when she came to see me and became pregnant within the first six weeks of Naturopathic care in our practice. I recall on her second visit explaining to her that even though she had been told she was infertile, she needed to be careful and conscious of contraception while she was undergoing treatment from myself. Little did we both know that day she was already pregnant and went on to have a beautiful baby girl.

I recall a male patient coming to me with a near zero sperm count. I offered him nutritional medicine and herbal supplements, adjusted and loosened his lower back to improve circulation to his prostrate and testes, along with advice on some improved dietary choices. He discovered his wife was pregnant on Father's Day only a few short months after.

Another one of my stand-out success stories was an 89-year-old patient suffering severe vomiting after eating any meal. She was slowly wasting away. I administered some iridology on that first consultation only to tell her she had gallstones, and she needed a flush. She was confused, saying her doctor said it was all clear. I recommended that she do the flush just in case to see what comes out.

To cut a long story short, she flushed thousands of small stones and went onto do several flushes, which completely resolved her vomiting. Her health then dramatically improved, as you can imagine, and she went on to live another 10 years in good health.

See RESOURCE 21: Liver and Gallbladder

A Running Commentary

There's a wonder drug called Epsom salts
That induces relaxation
So I took of it quite liberally
And here's an explanation

When I joined the Epsom Derby
It was my darkest hour
'Cause it caused a situation
Over which I had no power

The Flying Nun had naught on me
As I flew towards the Loo
And if you'd taken what I had
You'd do the same thing too!

Back & forth I trotted
With the speed of a startled gazelle
And how many miles an hour I went
I do not care to tell.

Down the hall I'd hurtle,
To hasten not, I durst
If I didn't make it just in time
I could expect the worst.

That I would be a winner,
I could tell it in my bones,

'Cause the prize for which I raced
Was many precious stones

They're not the little nuggets
You would pan for in the River
But the green stones that are lodging
In an organ called the liver.

I had a competition
With daughter Chris to see
Who could run the fastest
It wasn't her — 'twas me!!

This is the end of my tale about Epsom,
Though it caused me some commotion
But, for the purpose of removal
Its really quite a potion.

by Viola
26-10-95

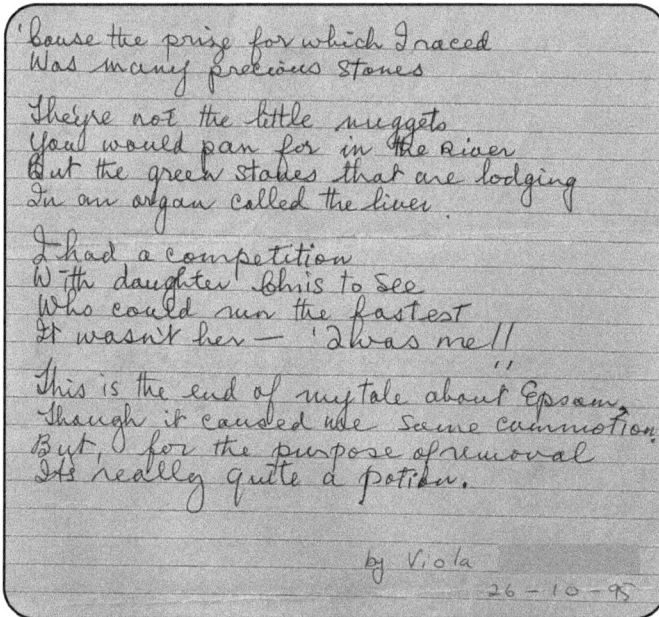

A more recent story is a 16-year-old patient that was experiencing a complete deterioration of her health. She had been very healthy all her life and I had consulted the family for years with natural medicine for colds, coughs, spinal care, and menstrual care, all with good results. But by the time she came in, I had not consulted with her for a few years because she had been well and healthy, or so I thought. She walked into the room very slowly and her movements were also very timid. She reported that she had not had a menstrual cycle for months and was overall very introverted, quiet, and nervous, with acne breakout on her face.

I was shocked as this was quite the opposite from her usual extroverted, bright, bubbly, personality I remembered. At first, she responded well and got her menstrual cycle back; her movement seemed better and there was a little improvement in her demeanour.

However, this phase did not last, and she deteriorated before my very eyes over the next months. I sent her for medical testing and by now was sure she had a neurological inflammation of her brain. It took four doctors and a stint in the Royal Children's Hospital to even get her basic physical tests done, but even they could not find out what was wrong with her.

The medical professionals just wanted to label her with a mental illness. I was unconvinced that her symptoms were not of a physical nature, and with the gallantry her parents showed, they persisted with her tests until finally we had a diagnosis: PANDAS, an infection that enters the brain via the sinuses.

We continued to treat her for brain inflammation and infection, and we are now seeing a gradual but definite improvement. The treatment, apart from antibiotics (both natural and medical and a powerful anti-inflammatory liquid curcumin), has made the difference. But the biggest change came with some of my energy medicine: creating healing energy and putting it into her brain, nervous system, and connecting her CNS to her bladder and bowel again. She had lost all control of both bodily functions in those prior few months. She is now able to take herself to the bathroom once again and her parents are diligently giving her all the correct nutrients to nourish her inflamed brain.

This young lady was one of the toughest cases I have ever had to confront, and it takes a front seat with that of my granddaughter who was diagnosed with leukaemia at nine months old. She has just turned nine years old today as I write this.

When this was discovered, my granddaughter was given a prognosis of only a 30% survival rate or any chance of recovery. She had presented with a severe aggressive form of leukaemia, rarely seen in children, let alone a baby. But with the help of the Royal Children's Hospital here in Melbourne, and a lot of natural medicine including NAET (allergy elimination treatment), herbs, vitamins, minerals, and probiotics, she not only survived but has gone on to be one of the brightest and happiest little girls you could ever meet.

We did one other very important thing while she was having treatment. We organised a spiritual counsellor from our religion to assist her with a gentle technique developed especially for leukaemia in children. I fully believe we saved her life using all three modalities at once: allopathic medicine,

Naturopathic medicine, and spiritual counselling. We also decided on a policy to never let anyone cry in front of her or show sympathy of the type that drives a person into grief. We only discussed her case and its severity away from her, so she was not frightened by the thought of pending death and failure. We had music, creative art, and anything good that children love around her at all times.

As a family, we learned a lot from her. She would handle the repeated blood tests like it was a normal thing and held her arm out with no drama at all. She was brave and showed courage at all times. She would immediately be happy as long as she was not in pain. She would let go of anything that was painful, harmful, or dramatic, and would be fully in the present, and looking toward her future continually.

Even her perception was amazing. If I was with her, and her mum or dad walked into the hospital to see her, she immediately knew and would say "Mamma is here; Dada is here." I would look at my watch and think, yeah maybe. And sure enough, she was right every time. She would also predict the weather and say "Wet coming." I would say, "You mean rain?" And she would nod. I would look outside and it would be sunny, but sure enough, within the hour – it would be raining. To this day I still don't know how she knew this at the age of one. But she did.

There is so much to life we don't yet understand, but it can be miraculous and amazing and full of love and life, with so much out there to help you.

If you are a person suffering from a condition and have all but given up hope of receiving some form of guidance, treatment, or help – don't. Keep looking. Your answer will come if you are persistent and keep in your mind a picture of yourself well, healthy, and pain-free.

Conclusion

Something has led mankind to spending more and more money on drugs today than food. More and more people are dependent upon drugs to relieve their ailments, escape boredom, and prop up their ability to face the day. Even children now take drugs and millions are given sedatives and amphetamines in the classroom all over the world. What has changed in our attitudes about dealing with existence to the point where we just rub a chemical salve on every part of life?

Below is from the Australian Institute of Child Health and Welfare.

Prescription drug use increased with age, overall and among males and females. Overall, 18.0% of children aged 0–11 years, 27.0% of adolescents aged 12–19, 46.7% of adults aged 20–59, and 85.0% of adults aged 60 and over used prescription drugs in the past 30 days.

Undoubtedly, the change has come from within mankind itself. Something, whatever it is, has affected the way in which we think and the way in which we behave. The subjects within this book contain help, advice, and suggestions on what you can do right now, right here to begin a new change of mind, and thereby, regain a new level of health.

Physical health, which is the basis for mental, emotional, and spiritual development, cannot be maintained without adequate nutrition. This is your fortress against disease and this strength protects you and those you love. Forget about your age: balance your life, balance your activities, balance your emotions, balance your relationships, and, most importantly, balance your diet.

It is my sincerest hope that this book will contribute to the enhancement of the physical, emotional, and spiritual wellbeing of anyone seeking truth, and a complete wholistic approach to life, happiness, and good health.

Intelligence on a cellular level, which controls cellular discipline, reproduction, growth, and development, aids repair of wear and tear of our body, must be tuned into.

Listen to your body and acknowledge the warning bells. Be proactive and do what you know to be right for you and your body. Push through all the reasons why you feel you should *not* do something beneficial for yourself and your body, and do what you intuitively KNOW to be the right thing to do for you!

You have it within you to respond constructively and creatively to anything and everything that is taking place in your life. I believe in miracles; I have seen miracles; I believe in you too!

At first, change may feel startling, refreshing, or even disruptive. It may be welcomed warmly or contemplated cautiously. Yet, change can be a wake-up call, providing you with a path that has become clear in your own journey to wellness.

For me and my personal journey, helping others, the more the better, has kept a fire burning within me all these years. As a result of the love for my work, I will continue teaching and healing others for as long as I breathe. Never will I give up on this: it is my driving, burning passion and unrelenting purpose in life.

I would love to hear from those of you who have undertaken some of the principles in this manuscript, as this would be my greatest reward.

Yours in health,

Love Nerida

Dr Nerida James
ND. DC Dip Irid Cert Hom.

Success Stories

4 January, 1999

Dear Nerida,

I have been seeing you for approximately 15 months now, and I would like to let you know how much my health has improved in that time.

The main reason I made the first appointment was because I was desperate to get rid of my acne, and you were highly recommended by one of your clients. Since following the acid and alkaline food diet, combined with regular exercise, my skin has greatly improved. I have fewer cravings for lollies and biscuits, and combined with the diet and exercise I have lost 7 kilos (I even managed to keep it off over Christmas!). My energy levels have also increased dramatically.

My curvature of the spine also seems to have decreased, and regular manipulation has decreased the number of headaches caused by it, and improved my flexibility.

Thanks for all your help in improving my health Nerida, and I look forward to even more benefits this year!

Sincerely,

Lisa

Success Story

15·9·95

Nerida,

thank-you very much for helping me clear the skin condition on my hand. Unsuccessfully, I contacted a doctor who put me on penicillin for a week - after finishing the script, my infection reappeared. Nerida gave me a natural anti-biotic which helped clear my infection (in the form of a Golden Stuff) within days. Together with homeopathic Thuja cream my infected hand now looks normal again. I was surprised that natural products could clear my hand so successfully & so quickly and, there were no side effects experienced. I never expected my hand to clear so rapidly. Thanks again,

Andrea.

SUCCESS STORY   25-5-2011

I hadn't been feeling well for a couple of months, so I went to see my GP. She diagnosed me with anxiety & exhaustion & prescribed me anti-depressants; referred me to a Physcologist. The tablets weren't helping & I didn't think the physcologist was either, I still felt the same. My girlfriend then referred me to see Nerida. Nerida pretty much summed me up in 5 minutes on my 1st visit. Alcohol was the problem that had been causing my anxiety. I had never been a big drinker, but I must say the last 5 years I have been drinking wine 7 nights a week. I thought it was ok to do that; that it was ok; good for you to drink everyday. 5 o'clock everynight the TV would come on; out comes the wine glass as I prepare tea. I was having at least 3 a night. Nerida worked this out to be 4500 alcohol drinks in 5 years after doing my urology. Nerida said I had inflamed kidneys, liver, pancreas; that I needed to stop what I had been doing. Nerida told me to stop the alcohol, sugar; she put me on vitamins. I have been taking my vitamins everyday & only have a glass of wine as a treat on a Friday or Saturday night. Its amazing how good I feel without the alcohol. I'm not clouded by it, I'm more alert & can make rational decisions. I felt as though my head was clouded & now my head feels like blue sky with no clouds, its an amazing feeling, I absolutely feel like a new woman. I will never drink alcohol during the week again, its not ok, you think it is, but it only makes you depressed. I feel FANTASTIC! I love taking my vitamins. Nerida I dearly thank you from the bottom of my heart for your genuine care in my health & for your passion in believing in Natural healing.

        love, health & happiness forever

        Tania

        X O X

January 2006.

Thankyou Nerida,

When my son Jy was 2 weeks old he started to show the signs on severe gastric reflux. For 6 months we were baffled by the medical profession and told that 'eventually' Jy would grow out of it. In the meantime, however, we were expected to give him @ 3 different drugs, 4 times a day and whilst it seem to stop the pain and help us all sleep, it was clear that he wasn't healthy.

Finally, we bowed to a friends pressure and made our first visit to you.

You cured Jy almost instantly (it took a couple of weeks to wean him off the drugs) and the transformation was miraculous!

Jy is now a normal - extremely healthy - 10 year old. I will continue to recommend you to anyone and everyone, and I could never thank you enough for what you have given Jy

Julie

My name is Lucy, on the 18TH APRIL 1998 I experienced the worst pain on my left side you can imagine. For the next few weeks I spent in and out of hospital for scans, xrays, medications and intensive screening almost on a daily basis. Finally after many worrying and sleepless nights it was diagnosed I had a growth the size of a small fist on my liver and where it is situated is not easily accessible if an operation was an option. Through talking with friends and family we were told about Dr. NERIDA JAMES. She has brought me back to being healthier than I have felt in many years, the growth has shrunk, I have more energy and vibrancy and my family and myself are extremely grateful.

Thank You NERIDA
Lucy and family

Dear Nerida,

Thank you so much for all of your help and support over the past year.

I definatly wouldn't be competing in the Commenweatlth Games this March if it wasn't for everything you have done for me.

Once Again, thankyou for all your hard work!

Love Ashleigh xox

She is 10 years old and just 135cm tall but Melissa Taylor is a name that everyone will know before to long! This extraordinary young lady from Mooroolbark has the poise and maturity of someone twice her age, is already a very accomplished golfer and one of the two youngest members of Chirnside Park Country Club.

Things have not been easy for Melissa who, at only eighteen months of age, became painfully ill with severe muscle weakness. The doctors at the Royal Children's' Hospital in Melbourne diagnosed her condition as Dermatomyositis, an autoimmune disease that affects about one in eight hundred thousand people. After leaving hospital, her parents Mark and Kathy, set about helping their daughter on the long road to recovery. With the knowledge that intensive physiotherapy was the ideal treatment, they introduced Melissa to a range of physical games that would help her to regain the strength in her muscles.

When she was three, Santa Claus paid her a visit and left a set of plastic golf clubs.

Toy clubs lasted no time at all in the hands of this amazing girl and she quickly graduated to more serious tools, an old cane 2 Iron and a cut down 7 *Iron*.

Coached by her father, she practised in her back garden but was forced to move to more open spaces as her swing developed and at 5yrs of age she could drive a golf ball 50mts and straight as a die!

She has been in remission since 1997 and Melissa is now hooked on the game that she claims has helped her back to health.

Last year, Melissa became a member of the Chirnside Park Country Club and a member of Women's Golf Victoria with a special invitation to the Young Tyro's program for elite golfers with the institute of sport at the Melbourne Golf Academy.

One of the highlights in her life was meeting and getting to know Karrie Webb who has become her idol.

With Karrie's encouragement, Melissa now has her sights set on a professional golf career.

During the Rotary Club of Croydon's 15th annual golf day, Melissa added to her impressive list of trophies when she took honours for the longest ladies drive for the afternoon, the best Stableford for lady handicap players with a score of 47 points playing off 36 and was part of the winning foursome that scored 39.66 points.

Publication 2007

Swinging like a star

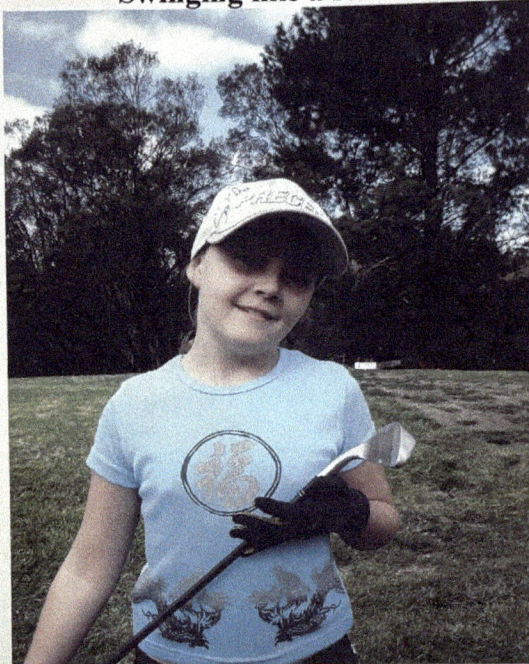

Melissa has been a patient of Dr. Nerida James at the Natural Healing centre in Mitcham for the past 6 months, in this time the progress Melissa has shown on the path to good health has been impressive she has grown 10cm and gained 9kgs.

This has given her more stamina and strength in the pursuit of her dream.

Melissa attends Bimbadeen Heights Primary; she enjoys art, music and twice has represented the school in chess competitions.

Melissa lists tennis, Karate, Swimming and playing pool amongst her other sporting interests.

To Nerida,
Thanks for all your help so far you've been great for me.
Love
Melissa. T.

18. 3. 93.

DEAR NERIDA,
JUST A FEW WORDS OF THANKS TO YOU FOR MY RECENT TREATMENT BY YOURSELF, TO MY JAW. FOLLOWING REMOVAL OF A WISDOM TOOTH IN HOSPITAL, MY JAW BECAME STIFF AND PAINFUL TO MOVE. ON VISITING MY DENTIST HE ADVISED ME I WAS SUFFERING FROM 'DOFOS' WHICH IS A DISTURBANCE OF FUNCTIONAL OCCLUSION SYNDROME, TREATING WITH MANY VISITS AND FITTING AN OVERLAY DENTURE WAS ADVISED, AT A COST OF ₿1350 UPWARDS.
MY TWO VISITS TO NERIDA AT A COST OF ₿75, NOT ONLY SAVED ME ₿1275, BUT WEARING A DENTURE FOR THE REST OF MY LIFE.
ONCE AGAIN MY SINCERE THANKS.
YOURS FAITHFULLY
D.

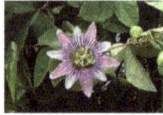

Herbal Tonics – Nerida's Elixirs

C-Hox tonic (500ml)

Liquorice – 75ml

Red Clover – 75ml

Burdock Root – 50ml

Queen's Delight – 50ml

Poke Root – 25ml

Cascara – 50ml

Prickly Ash – 25ml

Barberry – 50ml

Buckthorn Bark – 25ml

Cleavers (clivers) – 75ml

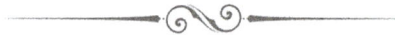

Prostate Tonic (200ml)

Equal Parts – 28.5ml per herb

Saw palmetto

Pau d'arco

Ginseng

Damiana

Sarsaparilla

Oats

Schizandra

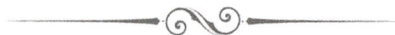

Adrenal Tonic (200ml)

Withania – 30ml

Siberian Ginseng – 20ml

Rhodiola – 30ml

Panax Ginseng – 10ml

Liquorice – 10ml

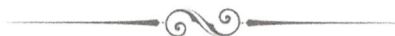

C-Hox: Alternate 1

Liquorice – 50ml

Red clover – 75ml

Burdock root – 50ml

Turkey tail – 50ml

Poke root – 25ml

Cascara – 50ml

Gotu kola – 25ml

Barberry/Pau d'arco – 50ml

Buckthorn bark – 25ml

Cleavers – 50ml

Rhubarb – 50ml

Hayfever/Sinus tonic (200ml)

Astragalus – 20ml

Olive leaf – 35ml

Fennel – 25ml

Marshmallow – 25ml

Liquorice – 25ml

Gotu Kola – 20ml

Yarrow – 25ml

Hawthorn berries – 25ml

Adhesion/ Scar tissue tonic:

Equal Parts:

Calendula

Dan Shen

Comfrey

Gotu Kola

Energy tonic (200ml bottle)

Ginseng – 40ml

Sarsaparilla – 30ml

Withania – 40ml

Astragalus – 30ml

Liquorice – 30ml

Nettle – 30ml

———— ❧ ————

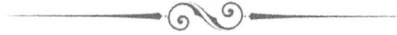

Lymph tonic (200ml bottle – equal parts)

Cleavers – 33.3ml

Yellow Dock – 33.3ml

Pau d'arco – 33.3ml

Poke root – 33.3ml

Echinacea – 33.3ml

Goldenseal – 33.3ml

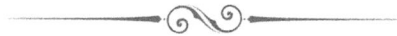

———— ❧ ————

Bowel tonic (for reducing scars) (200ml bottle – equal parts)

Comfrey – 50ml

Calendula – 50ml

Gotu Kola – 50ml

Dan shen – 50ml

———— ❧ ————

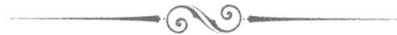

Tooth & gum formula (2 x 50ml bottles)

Cayenne – 4ml

Oak bark – 25ml

Barberry – 25ml

Echinacea – 45ml

Clove oil – 1ml (20 drops)

Tea tree oil – 2ml (30 drops)

Peppermint oil – 2ml (30 drops)

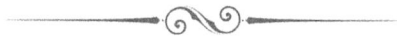

———— ❧ ————

CelluFree Blood tonic (200ml – equal parts)

Kelp – 20ml

Liquorice – 20ml

Uva Ursi – 20ml

Juniper berries – 20ml

Parsley leaf – 20ml

Chickweed – 20ml

Hawthorn – 20ml

Dandelion – 20ml

Burdock – 20ml

Papaya fruit – 20ml

Blood cleanser (200ml – equal parts except chlorophyll)

Dandelion – 47.5ml

Burdock – 47.5ml

Red Clover – 47.5ml

Sarsaparilla – 47.5ml

Chlorophyll – 10ml

Phyto formula: Female (200ml bottle)

Dong quai – 30ml

Ginger – 10ml

Black cohosh – 40ml

Peonia – 20ml

False unicorn – 30ml

Cramp bark – 20ml

Blue cohosh – 30ml

Wild yam – 20ml

Liver tonic (200ml bottle)

Globe artichoke – 28.5ml

Celandine (Chelidonium) –18.5ml

Yellow dock – 28.5ml

Red clover – 28.5ml

Dandelion – 28.5ml

Liquorice – 28.5ml

St Mary's thistle – 38.5ml

Detox tonic (200ml bottle – equal parts)

Burdock – 28.5ml

Sarsaparilla – 28.5ml

Red clover – 28.5ml

Oak bark – 28.5ml

Rhubarb root – 28.5ml

Nettle – 28.5ml

Chlorophyl – 28.5ml

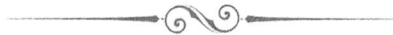

Polycystic ovaries (200ml bottle – equal parts)

Liquorice 1:1 or 1:2 – 22.2ml

Paeonia – 22.2ml

Saw palmetto – 22.2ml

Hops – 22.2ml

Black cohosh – 22.2ml

Sarsaparilla – 22.2ml

Chaste tree – 22.2ml

Korean ginseng – 22.2ml

Sage or false unicorn – 22.2ml

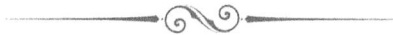

Resco-bronchial formula (equal parts)

Liquorice

Mullein

Euphorbia

Grindelia

Elecampane

Ginger

Fennel

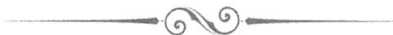

Herbal immune tonic (20ml = 200ml bottle – equal parts)

Echinacea

Ginseng

Cleavers

Nettle

Red clover

Liquorice

Astragalus

Olive leaf

Propolis

Chlorophyll (for taste)

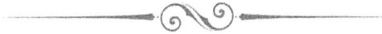

3-in-1 Herbs – Parasite cleanse

50% Black walnut

25% Cloves

25% Wormwood

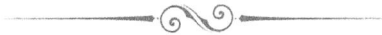

2-in-1 Herbs (for those allergic to wormwood or pregnant women)

50% Black Walnut

50% Cloves

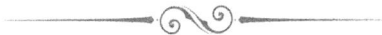

Hep-C Herbs for eliminating hep-C

2 bags of herbs, 12 grams of each herb boiled together with 3 to 4 cups of water and simmer down to a cup and drink all at once, one cup a day till necessary.

2 Herbs:

- Ban zhi lian (portulaca grandiflora)

- Bai hua she cao (hedyotis diffusa)

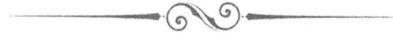

Yeasts – Anti-fungal tonic (200ml bottle)

St Mary's thistle – 80ml

Echinacea – 40ml

Pau d'arco – 50ml

Goldenseal – 10ml

Black walnut – 20ml

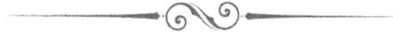

Progesterone tonic (200ml bottle)

Wild yam – 50ml

Chaste tree – 50ml

Dong quai – 40ml

Black cohosh – 35ml

Lady's mantle – 25ml

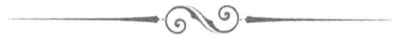

Pain relief tonic (200ml bottle)

Boswellia – 30ml

Rosemary – 50ml

Hops – 40ml

Olive leaf – 40ml

Rosehips – 40ml

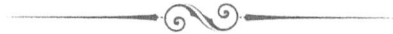

Period pain tonic

Chaste tree – 25%

Cramp bark – 50%

Blue cohosh 25%

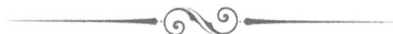

Infection fighter
(200ml bottle)

Blue flag – 40ml

Propolis – 10ml

Echinacea – 50ml

Goldenseal – 50ml

Olive leaf – 50ml

Antiviral tonic (200ml bottle)

Maritime pine – 40ml

Arjuna – 20ml

Turmeric – 40ml

Dandelion – 20ml

Green tea – 20ml

Elecampane – 20ml

Andrographis – 20ml

Ginger – 20ml

Immune-boosting tonic

Olive leaf – 30%

Propolis – 10%

Echinacea – 20%

Astragalus – 15%

Andrographis – 15%

Marshmallow – 10%

Menopause tonic
(200ml bottle)

Rehmannia – 50ml

Chaste tree – 40 ml

Paeonia – 50ml

Ziziphus – 30ml

St John's Wort – 10ml

Siberian rhubard – 20ml

Oestrogen-lift tonic
(200ml bottle; 20ml each)

Rehmannia

Wild yam

Peony root & bark

Plantain

Black cohosh

Liquorice

Damiana

Chaste tree

Alfalfa

Lady's mantle

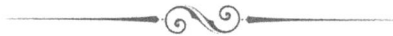

Stop smoking tonic
(equal parts, 25ml each)

Valerian

Skullcap

Blue cohosh

Black cohosh

Peppermint

Slippery elm

Poke root (phytolacca)

Chlorophyll (for taste)

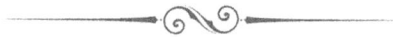

Female tonic (equal parts; 25ml each)

Pulsatilla

Ginseng

Lady's mantle

Dong quai

Chaste tree

Blue cohosh

Black cohosh

Sarsaparilla

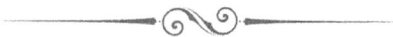

Fibroid tonic (475ml; equal parts; 47.5ml each)

Chaste tree

Sarsaparilla

Thuja

Raspberry

Wild yam

Black cohosh

Chelidonium

Dong quai

St Mary's thistle

Dandelion root

Poke root – 25ml

Chronic cough mix (200ml bottle)

Ivy leaf (Hedera helix) – 20ml

Echinacea – 40ml

Elecampane – 30ml

Liquorice – 40ml

Thyme – 30ml

Grindelia – 28ml

Euphorbia – 10ml

Peppermint oil – 3 drops

Herbal cough mixture (200ml bottle)

Echinacea – 25ml

Thyme – 25ml

Peppermint – 25ml

Mullein – 25ml

Marshmallow – 25ml

White horehound – 25ml

Liquorice – 25ml

Elecampane – 25ml

Arthrileaf (200ml bottle)

Liquorice – 25ml

Celery seed – 50ml

Feverfew – 25ml

Ginger – 25ml

Marshmallow – 25ml

Comfrey – 50ml

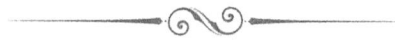

Kidney tonic (diuretic)
(200ml bottle; equal parts)

Juniper – 28.5ml

Dandelion – 28.5ml

Uva Ursi – 28.5ml

Celery – 28.5ml

Buchu – 28.5ml

Liquorice – 28.5ml

Shatavari (asparagus racemosus) – 28.5ml

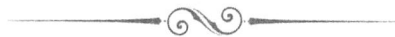

Testosterone-lowering tonic (200ml bottle; equal parts 50ml)

Liquorice

Chaste tree

Paeonia

Sage

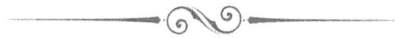

Milk stimulant tonic
(200ml bottle)

Fennel – 50ml

Chaste tree – 40ml

Fenugreek – 50ml

Alfalfa – 40ml

Nettle – 10ml

Ginger – 10ml

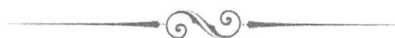

Circulation tonic – for lymph and cardiovascular (200ml bottle)

Gotu kola – 80ml

Witch hazel – 40ml

Hawthorn berries – 40ml

Ginkgo biloba – 20ml

Yarrow – 20ml

Fatty liver tonic (200ml bottle)

Schisandra – 20ml

Indian barberry – 20ml

Globe Artichoke – 20ml

Liquorice – 20ml

Celandine (Chelidonium) – 10ml

Yellow dock – 20ml

Red clover – 10ml

Dandelion – 20ml

St Mary's thistle – 60ml

Nerve/Sleep tonic (200ml bottle; equal parts 25ml)

Skullcap

Passionflower

Valerian

Chamomile

Oats

Ziziphus Jujuba

Magnolia

Lemon Balm

Candida tonic (200ml bottle; equal parts 25ml)

Chlorophyll

Juniper berries

Skullcap

Fucus

St Mary's thistle

Pau d'arco

Horopito

Dandelion

Laxative tonic (200ml bottle)

Cascara – 75ml

Liquorice – 50ml

Senna – 75ml

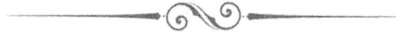

Eye tonic (200ml bottle)

Bilberry – 60ml

Eyebright – 60ml

Dandelion – 25ml

Chamomile – 30ml

Goldenseal – 25ml

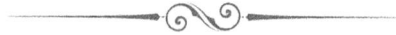

Indigestion tonic (200ml bottle; equal parts 25ml)

Juniper

Celery

Alfalfa

Liquorice

Peppermint oil – 3 drops

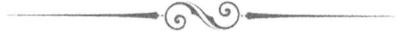

Pleurisy tonic (200ml bottle; equal parts 25ml)

Pelargonium

Pleurisy root

Hawthorn

Echinacea

Panax ginseng

Mullein

Lobelia

Marshmallow root

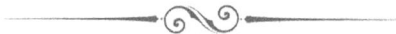

Anxiety tonic (200ml bottle)

Ziziphus – 40ml

Kava – 20ml

Lemon balm – 40ml

Magnolia – 40ml

Passion flower – 50ml

Lavender – 10ml

Pneumonia/ Bronchitis tonic (200ml bottle)

Houttuynia – 50ml

Ivy leaf – 50ml

Goldenseal – 30ml

Andrographis - 14ml

Japonica - 14ml

Boswellia - 14ml

Fennel - 14ml

Korean ginseng -14ml

Testosterone-boosting tonic (200ml bottle)

Tongkat ali glycerate – 75ml

Tribulus leaf – 85ml

Korean ginseng – 40ml

Resources

1. To sustain life – nothing lives without water

2. To generate electrical and magnetic energy

3. Acts as a bonding adhesive to cells

4. Prevents DNA damage

5. Makes tissue repair more efficient

6. Increases manifold the efficiency of the immune system

7. Is the main solvent of all foods

8. Is used in the breakdown of foods for metabolism

9. Energises food

10. Increases the rate of absorption of food

11. Is used for transfer of all substances in the body

12. Clears the toxic wastes from the body

13. Brings oxygen to the cells

14. Is the main lubricant in the joint spaces

15. Is a laxative and prevents constipation

16. Prevents heart attacks and strokes

17. Is used to cushion spinal discs (back pain can occur when dehydrated)

18. Prevents clogging of the arteries in the heart

19. Is essential in the cooling and heating of the body

20. Operates a two-way heat pump for summer and winter heat

21. Gives power for brain function – thinking

22. Prevents attention deficit disorders in children and adults

23. Is the best single "pick me up" beverage with no side-effects

24. Prevents depression, stress, anxiety

25. Will restore normal sleep rhythm

26. Prevents fatigue

27. Makes skin smooth and prevents aging

28. Gives lustre and shine to the eyes

29. Maintains vision

30. Prevents glaucoma

31. Dilutes blood and prevents clotting during circulation

32. Decreases premenstrual pains

33. Prevents sedimentation in the bloodstream

34. Promotes sex hormone production

35. Decreases likelihood of sexual impotence

36. Decreases libido

37. Takes away morning sickness when pregnant

38. Integrates mind and body function

39. Reverses addictive urges including caffeine and alcohol

The Drastic Indicators of Dehydration

A. Emotional

Feeling tired

Feeling anxious

Feeling irritable

Feeling dejected, insufficient, inadequate

Feeling depressed

Having a heavy head, slight headache

Disturbed sleep

Anger and quick temper

Unreasonable impatience

Short attention span

Shortness of breath

Cravings for coffee, tea, sodas, and other manufactured beverages

B. Pain

Dyspeptic pain

Colitis pain

Hiatus Hernia pain

Rheumatoid arthritis pain

Lower back pain

Neck pain

Anginal pain

Headache pain

Intermittent claudication

Morning sickness

Bulimia

C. Disease States

- Hypertension
- Asthma
- Allergies
- Raised cholesterol
- Heart failure
- Diabetes
- Repeated strokes

- Alzheimer's disease
- Multiple sclerosis
- Cancers
- Coronary thrombosis
- Plaque build-up in major arteries

RESOURCE 2 : My Healthy Diet Sheet

BREAKFAST: Fruit juice only preferred. If hungry, eat fresh fruit, fruit salad, or chia pods. Organic or biodynamic Greek, soya, or coconut yoghurt may be eaten twice/three times weekly. An excellent cereal combination is puffed millet, puffed rice, rolled oats, sesame seeds, sunflower seeds, barley flakes, and rice flakes, all of which would be available from your local health food store. Millet or buckwheat could be boiled with water or soy milk to make porridge. Buckwheat pancakes with organic maple syrup, lemon juice, and sugar-free jam on toast can be eaten. NOTE: Gluten-free wheatbix (sorghum), cereals, breads, and cow's milk yoghurt are acid and mucus-forming and should only be eaten two to three times per week. Cow's milk and cheese should be avoided, especially for those with sinus issues or hay fever.

LUNCH: Fresh salads including alfalfa, celery, parsley, fresh basil, lettuce, tomato, spring onions, grated carrot, beetroot, roquette, or baby spinach. Also, almonds and cashews should be included. Sandwiches using salad ingredients with organic (yeast-free) sourdough breads. Many breads have synthetic folic acid, mold inhibitors (Penicillin), plus other added chemicals such as artificial yeasts and preservatives. Crispbreads – rice cakes, cruskits; rye, buckwheat, corn, sweet potato, chestnut with hummus, tahini, or avocado spreads, tomato, sprouts – anything healthy and fresh will do. Use your imagination! Vegetable soups, including pumpkin, leek, mixed veggies and barley, celery, tomato, etc, using yeast-free, stock cubes (no MSG) or bone broth with lots of herbs and spices for flavour. Always include a green leafy vegetable in your soups such as parsley, basil, silver beet, spinach, or carrot tops. Baked potatoes in their jackets with salads are also a good winter lunch with soup.

SNACKS/DRINKS: Whole grain snacks including biscuits/muffins (almond flour and gluten free with sweeteners such as stevia, xylitol, or monk fruit in cakes), celery or carrot sticks with hummus or avocado dip, rice cakes or cruskits with cashew nut spread or ABC spread (almond, brazil, cashew). Nuts – activated and lightly salted. Water is preferably filtered. Mineral or spring water are available bottled. Coffee substitutes: Caro, cacao, dandelion, and others. Herb teas: peppermint, rosehip, lemongrass, spearmint are a few favourites; maybe sweetened with agave or coconut sugar, xylitol, or mānuka honey. Unsalted or low salt butter is recommended in moderation as margarine is a toxic oil that does not occur naturally. Almond milk can be made easily or can be purchased from most supermarkets, as can oat milk. Coconut organic yoghurt and chia pods are also a great snack.

DINNER: Grassfed meats, hormone-free chicken, and wild-caught fish three times weekly (or more if there is a heavy physical workload), free range eggs – 4 per week (quiche, omelette, etc). Pasta dishes twice weekly using only wholemeal, buckwheat, rye, spelt, amaranth, rice, or millet. Sauces can include a vegetable base, such as tomato and herb, also a creamy sauce using coconut cream and garlic. Stir fry vegetables using cold-pressed oil. Add finely grated ginger, crushed garlic and onion, olive oil, avocado oil, etc, then add vegetables in order of the longest time to cook to shortest time to cook. Add tamari soy sauce one minute prior to serving and toss veggies continuously. Vegetable pies or pasties, using wheat-free pastry only. Tofu or tempeh (soy protein) can be cut into cubes or thick strips and fried in cold-pressed oil until golden brown and drain on paper towels or marinated and baked in the oven, serve with or without a bed of brown rice, topped with a healthy sauce.

Long grain brown rice dishes are a good source of B vitamins and protein (or organic basmati white rice for those with sensitive digestion) and may be eaten once a week or more. Legumes, lentils, beans, and chickpeas may be used in stir-fry or veggie casseroles (best pressure-cooked). Tacos with beans and salad.

NOTE: Try to use as much garlic, onion, and herbs in your cooking (unless otherwise advised) and always have a tossed salad or veggies as an accompaniment to your meal. Locally grown, organic vegetables are preferable and nutritionally superior to regular fruit and veggies. Vegetarian and keto cookbooks are a great source of cooking ideas and inspiration.

ALTERNATIVES: Plant-based ice cream or coconut cream instead of cream, balsamic vinegar or lemon juice and cold-pressed oil salad dressing. Soy, rice, rye, or millet flour for thickening gravies or stews. When making healthy desserts can use agar agar, arrowroot, or kudzu as thickeners. Tahini (sesame seed paste) is the highest food source of calcium and is a key ingredient of hummus dip.

This diet should have healthy fats (and be low in salt if you have high blood pressure) with approximately half the food consumed raw in the form of vegetables, salads, and fruits. Steaming, grilling, and baking are the best cooking methods. It is necessary to chew your food adequately. Drinks should be at least half an hour to an hour later after eating. Drink lots of water as this helps eliminate toxins via your kidneys. Avoid sweets, processed foods, processed cow's milk, artificial flavourings and colourings, chemicals, preservatives, and pesticides.

Please remember that the Paleo diet is one of the healthiest diets around, and it is what we have followed for many millions of years. The newly added items to our diet are the grains which have been eaten only for a few thousand years and most of our intolerances and allergic reactions are related to the newly added items in some of the grains (wheat) and dairy products, food additives, colourings, and artificial preservatives. Fresh is best. Soon you will learn to appreciate and love the principles involved in this diet. It will become second nature, and not only will you feel terrific, but you will also experience satiety and the enjoyment of eating healthy food. Please do not forget to take the supplements recommended as part of your program. Regular exercise is important, as is a restful sleep of 7 to 8 hours.

Shopping List:

• Toothpaste: mineral toothpaste	• Cold-pressed oil, coconut oil, olive oil
• Soy milk, rice milk, or almond milk (no added vegetable oils)	• Fruit and veggies: organic, where possible
	• Organic butter, wild-caught fish
• Raw nuts: cashews, almonds, etc	• Organic brown rice
• Tahini, tamari (wheat-free)	• Free-range eggs, chicken, grassfed meats.
• Yeast-free stock cubes, bone broth	• Sugar-free jam, nut spreads
• Organic coconut yoghurt, chia pods	• Herb teas

RESOURCE 3: My Sleep Hygiene Resource Sheet

Promotes sleep	Prevents sleep
• Go to bed and get up at same time.	• Going to bed when not tired.
• Have an early, light dinner.	• Coffee and chocolate after dinner.
• Comfortable mattress and bedding.	• Stress and anxiety.
• Read a book in bed.	• Poor-quality bedding.
• Relaxation exercises.	• Hot bedroom with no ventilation.
• Low light or blocking blue light at night.	• Using interactive devices at night.
• Time spent in nature, particularly in the afternoon.	• Bright light/blue light at night.
	• Indoors all day, no exercise.

Diet:

- Opt for a nutrient-rich, wholefood diet, inclusive of high intake of fruits and vegetables, lean protein, quality essential fatty acids, and wholegrains (limiting starchy grains and vegetables), with low intake of sugar/refined foods.

- Reduce caffeine, alcohol, and/or tobacco late in the day, particularly during the evening.[82]

- Time-restricted feeding has shown promising benefits in improving metabolic parameters, including sleep.[83]

- Extending caloric intake over the course of 15 hours can cause circadian rhythm disruption.

- Eat within a 6-to-11-hour window, ideally after sunrise and before sunset.[84]

- Avoid heavy meals at night, but consider a light snack before bed such as toast or a handful of nuts. This may prevent night-time waking due to hunger.[85]

- Reduce liquids in the last 4 hours before bedtime to prevent night-time urination.[86]

Lifestyle:

- Support circadian rhythm by addressing excessive light exposure and increasing daytime light exposure:

  - Avoid screens for at least 1 hour before bed (television, laptops, computers, tablets, smart phones).

  - Use eye masks and/or black out curtains while sleeping.

  - Glasses that block blue light may prevent the effects of blue light on melatonin production and are indicated for people who use interactive devices in the evening.[87]

Alternatively, blue light filter apps or settings can be installed/activated on devices to minimise blue light exposure.

  - Increase daytime exposure to natural light in addition to limited night light exposure.[88]

  - Spend at least 30 minutes outside with sunlight on the skin in the morning, i.e. this could be sunrise, between 11.00 am or 1.00 pm and twilight.

- Increase daytime activity, but avoid exercise within 3 to 5 hours of bedtime to prevent evening overstimulation.[89]
- Consider white and pink noise as a background sound for the sleep environment.[90]
  - White noise creates a constant ambient sound that helps to mask other noises, such as traffic.
  - Pink noise is similar to white noise; however, it is slightly louder and more powerful at the lower frequencies (i.e. white noise with a stronger bass tone).
  - Listening to binaural beats may also enhance sleep.
    - Using headphones to listen to multiple sound frequencies at the same time (i.e. left ear receives a 300 hertz (Hz) tone and right ear receives a 280 Hz tone) allows the brain to process and absorb a low-frequency 10 Hz soundwave.
    - This in turn may slow brainwave activity, reducing arousal and thereby supporting sleep cycles.

Sleep Hygiene:

- Go to bed with a calm mind; try to resolve arguments or set a time earlier in the day to review problems and perhaps write down plans, solutions, or things to do.[91]
- Melatonin may be of great assistance in helping the body to resume a normal circadian rhythm or the sleep wake cycle. This can be sourced from the pharmacy.

Reference: Metagenics Institute

RESOURCE 4: Bowen Therapy

Congratulations, you have just received your first Bowen treatment. You have just taken the first steps towards natural health and assisting your body to heal itself.

For the next four days your body will be working hard to correct any imbalances that it has and will be cleansing, so drink lots of purified water. The Bowen will start to work on a different and more subtle level while you are asleep. Most of the corrections in your body will occur in the first 24 hours, but will continue throughout the first four days. We call this a "four-day healing crisis" in which your muscles and ligaments release and spinal correction occurs gradually.

The following are some guidelines to follow, which will aid your process of healing:

1. Please do not stay in a seated position on the day of treatment for longer than half an hour. Every half hour during you general day, take the time to stand up for a few minutes. This is vital so your spine can realign itself and the Bowen messages can come from the brain to do their work.

2. Please do not play sport for at least 24 hours after receiving a treatment. Dependent on the severity of your injury, it may be necessary to abstain for the whole week.

3. Drink between 4 and 5 glasses of water per day as this helps to flush the toxins out of your body. If you feel any nausea, this is not cause for concern as it is just the toxins being released from your system.

4. If you experience any pain different from what you already have, this is a positive sign that your body is starting to change back into its normal anatomical position. To ease any pain, WALK. Any sensation is only temporary and will only last for a few hours. Walking stimulates better circulation, aids lymphatic drainage of any toxins that may be accumulated in your muscles, and assists the spinal realignment.

5. For five days after your Bowen treatment, do not undergo any other energy work, eg massage, chiropractic, physio, reflexology, ultrasonic work, etc, as this will cancel out the gentle energy work that is occurring in your body.

6. For at least 12 hours after your Bowen treatment, do not have extended HOT baths or showers or use ice therapy. Warm baths or showers are OK.

7. If your condition is chronic, please do not give up easily as it may take that one extra treatment to turn the corner to your wellbeing. Remember your chronic condition didn't happen overnight.

8. Bowen is a completely safe, non-manipulative therapy where your body restores its own harmony. This does not work against the body but with the body, in its own time.

RESOURCE 5: Depression, Anxiety and Insomnia

Do you or anyone you know suffer from depression, anxiety, or insomnia?

Have you considered the role that nutrition plays in these common yet debilitating conditions?

There is a growing body of evidence that suggests ensuring adequate nutritional intake can help alleviate the symptoms of these conditions.

Nutrition, food intolerances, hormone imbalances, and brain hormones have a profound effect on one's emotions and nerve function if out of balance.

It is not widely understood that nutrition has a part to play in one's mental health. Yet there have been many studies done that indicate mental health conditions are caused by a combination of "physical" and "psychological" factors, and we now know that many physical factors can have a profound negative effect on mental health, contributing to and predisposing mental illness including anxiety, depression, ADHD, bipolar disorder, and even schizophrenia. Therefore, addressing and alleviating the physical contributing factors assists the person to address and handle the psychological aspect of the problem.

Correct nutrition is vital to health and wellbeing. All the organs in the body rely on the correct nutrients to function at their optimum levels. Nutrients (vitamins, minerals, fatty acids, amino acids, and glyconutrients) can increase or decrease the levels of important chemicals in the body as well as influencing hormonal balance, toxicity, immune function, inflammation, and the blood's coagulability.

A deficiency of any single nutrient can alter brain function and lead to depression, anxiety, and other mental disorders (Encyclopedia of Natural Medicine).

The brain is perhaps the most delicate organ in the body, using as much as 30% of all the energy we derive from food. Actually, the brain operates like a chemical factory that constantly produces dozens of neurotransmitters which act as messengers to start, continue, or stop biochemical processes. Certain of these neurotransmitters also influence our moods. The only raw materials for these processes are vitamins, minerals, amino acids, fatty acids, and other nutrients.

Emotional Disturbances and Biochemical Imbalance

Research has shown that biochemical imbalances occur in the body's nervous system and hormonal levels when there is emotional disturbance and distress.

Recurring patterns of a number of biochemical factors have been identified in individuals who report experiencing symptoms related to anxiety, depression, ADHD, eating disorders (anorexia and bulimia), and other mental or behavioural conditions.

For instance, common biochemical imbalances (including nutritional deficiencies) related to depression and anxiety which have been observed in clinical practice are:

- Decreased availability of neurotransmitters such as serotonin, dopamine, norepinephrine, GABA, and acetylcholine
- Increased levels of toxic neurochemicals
- Lower levels of magnesium, zinc, or potassium
- Deficient levels of vitamins such as B5, B6, B9 (Folic Acid), and B12

- Undersupply of key cofactors, eg amino acids

We also now know that there are four neurotransmitters (brain biochemicals that include hormones), which physically affect our frame of mind. When we have enough of all four, our emotions seem to be stable. These neurotransmitters are:

- **Dopamine (norepinephrine/epinephrine):** a hormone that is essential to the normal nerve activity of the brain. It acts as a natural energizer and mental focuser.

- **GABA:** an amino acid occurring in the central nervous system, associated with the transmission of nerve impulses. It acts as a natural sedative.

- **Endorphin:** a protein substance in the brain. It acts as a natural painkiller.

- **Serotonin:** an amino acid (amine) that works in brain chemistry. It acts as a natural mood stabiliser and sleep promoter.

Toxic substances and overloads also create biochemical imbalances, causing depression, and should be tested for if the depression is unexpected and without apparent reason. Additionally, the presence of heavy metals (lead, cadmium, mercury) can inhibit thyroid function. The thyroid produces hormones used to regulate blood calcium levels and the central nervous system. Prolonged organic or synthetic toxicity robs the body of nutrients.

Vitamin and mineral deficiencies have a key part to play. For instance, during stressful periods, the need for certain nutrients may increase and our body's stores can become depleted or toxic substances can leach certain nutrients from the body leaving a deficiency. Our regular food intake may be inadequate to combat what ails us. If a deficiency sets in, various illnesses can result.

Below is a list of certain vitamins, minerals, and amino acids with some of the clinical studies showing their effect on wellbeing:

- **Zinc:** Deficiency may cause anorexia, loss of libido, and fatigue, all of which suggest depression and respond to zinc replacement (Tasman Jones C. Zinc deficiency states. Adv Intern Med 26:97-114, 1980). Children with zinc deficiency are irritable, tearful, and sullen. They are not soothed by close body contact and recent disturbances. (Moynahan EJ. Zinc deficiency and disturbances of mood and visual behavior. Lancet I:91, 1976)

- **Folic Acid or B9:** Folate deficiency is associated with a wide variety of psychiatric symptoms including depression as well as with neurologic symptoms of weakness, numbness, stiffness, and spasticity, both with or without muscular atrophy (Howard JS Folate deficiency in psychiatric practice. Psychosomatics 16:112-115)

- **Vitamin B6:** Is commonly low in people who are depressed. This is particularly true in people taking birth control pills or oestrogen in any other form as oestrogen blocks the activity of B6. (Melvyn R. Werbach, M.D., Nutritional Influences on Mental Health 2nd Edition. Depression:234)

- **B12:** Early manifestations of B12 deficiency may include depression, generalised weakness, fatigue, indigestion, and diarrhoea. (Goodman KI, Salt WB 2nd. Vitamin B12 deficiency. Important new concepts in recognition. Postgrad Med 88(3): 147-50, 1990). Depression is common among patients with a vitamin

B12 deficiency syndrome (Melvyn R. Werbach, M.D., Nutritional Influences on Mental Health 2nd Edition. Depression:238).

- **Magnesium:** A critical mineral used in sending messages along the nerves. Mild deficiency is commonly associated with anxiety. (Seelig MS, Berger AR, Spieholz N.Latent tetany and anxiety, marginal Mg deficit and normocalcemia. Dis Nerv Sys 36:461-4, 1975.) Children with chronic magnesium deficits may be characterised by excessive fidgeting, anxious restlessness, psychomotor instability, and learning difficulties in the presence of a normal IQ (Durlach J. Clinical aspects of chronic magnesium deficiency, in MS Seelig, Ed. Magnesium in Health and Disease, New York, Spectrum Publications, 1980)

- **Amino acids:** Are the building blocks that make up protein. One form of the amino acid methionine is called SAMe. The most common reported effect of SAMe is mood elevation in depressed patients. (Spilman M, Fava M., S-Adenosylmethionine (Ademetionine) in psychiatric disorders: historical perspective and current status. CNS Drugs 6(6):416-25,1996.)

The good news is that toxic overloads and biochemical or hormonal imbalances (including nutritional deficiencies) can be identified through a combination of lab testing and examination of symptoms. Once found, the symptoms can be alleviated through appropriate natural treatment programs and nutritional supplementation.

The real cause of biochemical imbalance

Chemical imbalance is the latest popular theory to explain what causes mental illness. You may even have heard of this term. Put more precisely, the actual condition is a biochemical imbalance that affects the nervous system. This biochemical imbalance includes hormonal fluctuations and imbalance as part of its cause (produced by the endocrine system).

However, there is no proof that chemical or biochemical imbalance is the reason for mental illness. What does seem to be true is that biochemical and hormonal imbalances do occur and that these imbalances are formed as a result of our own thoughts and emotions.

Our behaviour and actions are governed by our thoughts and mental reactions to various stimuli. This gets processed through our nervous system of which the brain is a part. The central nervous system receives and interprets data. The brain initiates the body's responses by using neurotransmitters as messengers to start, continue, or stop certain activities.

It works like this:

You are heading home in your car, driving along on the freeway at 100km per hour. You hear screeching tyres and the car ahead of you breaks suddenly. Your mind immediately responds with a command for your foot to hit the brakes. Instantly, messages are sent and your foot slams on the brake pedal. At the same time, your brain rapidly releases neurotransmitters like norepinephrine which, in this situation, results in the production of adrenaline (a hormone). Your energy and mental acuteness instantly increase and you also start to feel nervous or tense. Your eyes widen; your palms begin to sweat; your heart is pounding. You command more action to be taken. Again, messages are sent; you check the rear vision mirror and swerve away from the car in front. You start to brace for impact. You are in a complete state of stress.

Luckily, your car misses the car that has stopped in front of you. As you pull over to the side of the road, you have a momentary feeling of disorientation and mild shock. You can't believe it. Your mind goes blank and you stare out the window. At this point, the brain redirects the blood and all the nutrients to the vital organs. Your hands start to tremble and you feel weak. To combat this, you force your attention outward and start to get angry. The brain again releases neurotransmitters to produce adrenaline and you get out of the car ready to do battle with the person who almost caused this accident.

However, you tell yourself to be calm and that the accident has been avoided. Your body feels tense, though, and you still feel nervous, so you take a deep breath and exhale. You tell yourself that you are lucky and your mood begins to lift. As you get back in your car and drive away, the chemicals in your brain begin to rebalance, hormones stop being produced, and along with the body's biochemistry, your thoughts eventually come back to a normal state.

This is an example of both the mind and body's immediate response to a perceived stressor. In the normal course of living, we encounter many different stressors. A stressor, by definition, must contain something that is counter to survival.

Our immediate response to a stressor involves all our senses and affects both mind and body. This becomes destructive to our mental and, subsequently, physical wellbeing only when the stressor(s) and the body's ensuing response(s) to them persist over time.

Suppose, for instance, in the above example, every time you drive somewhere and hear the screeching of breaks, your heart rate goes up and you begin to feel nervous. The nervous behaviour recurs so often that it begins to affect your outlook on driving and your response to other drivers also alters. Driving ceases to be a joy.

This is how behaviour and its physical response can become "wired in", causing a continual release of chemicals from the brain, triggering different responses in other parts of the body and depleting the body's overall nutritional reserves. As we make our way through life and more stressors accumulate, life becomes increasingly difficult and we experience feelings of exhaustion, anxiousness, irritability, or even depression.

Treating a biochemical or "chemical" imbalance

The medical community, with its emphasis on all things physical, has endorsed managing chemical imbalance through prescription drugs. But these drugs never truly correct the condition; they only alter or suppress the brain's chemistry. Once withdrawal is attempted, the condition comes back, often worse than before. The true condition stays in place because the drugs only target the chemical imbalance, which is an effect and not the underlying cause of the problem.

Additionally, synthetic drugs have been shown not to work in over half of cases and produce side-effects that may have both physical and mental repercussions of disastrous proportions. From my own clinical experience and observation in helping patients to withdraw off drugs, these medications cause such a suppression of the central nervous system that over the course of time higher doses or a mixture of drugs need to be given to achieve the same results. This in turn results in toxic overload and a downward spiral.

Which Doctor?

Of particular concern is that no one seems to know what the result of long-term psychotropic drug use will do to a person's health and longevity. From that perspective, this has all been one big experiment.

Compare this to a more natural and humane alternative that assists in handling the fundamental problem. Today, the knowledge that has been used to cure ills for thousands of years is backed up using modern scientific methods, while treatments and remedies still come in a form sympathetic to our own body's biological makeup. They do not have the same serious side-effects and, in many cases, are shown to be as or more effective. Nutritional supplementation is a valid form of treatment, with plenty of clinical studies to support this claim. However, addressing the mental factors that caused the physical problem to occur in the first place should also follow any physical treatment.

There are many options available these days. The first step is always to get informed.

Interesting websites:

- Safe Harbour: www.alternativementalhealth.com
  Interesting website with heaps of information and articles on different natural alternatives to mental health problems.

- Anxiety and Depression Solutions: www.anxiety-and-depression-solutions.com
  See articles on alternative medicine and health

- Health Research Institute & Pfeiffer Treatment Centre: www.hriptc.org
  A non-profit medical treatment & research organization that specializes in nutrient therapy for biochemical imbalances.

- Holistic Living: www.1stholistic.com
  Go to Nutrition, Vitamin & Diet Infocentre. Simple and informative.

- Narconon:
  An effective and comprehensive program for getting rid of toxic chemicals, radiation and drugs from the body.

Recommended Reading:

- *Say Good-bye to Illness* (3rd Edition), Dr Devi S Nambudripad, D.C., L.Ac., R.N., Ph.D.

The purpose of this information sheet is to inform patients there are natural antibiotics which can be more effective than the synthetic medical antibiotics for common infections.

The following paragraphs briefly describe some less well-known remedies. Medical antibiotics can be lifesaving in special circumstances but should be used sparingly and only on the advice of a specialist or MD.

Propolis

For many years, we have used a little-known remedy called propolis as an effective antibiotic made by the bees. It is a substance the bees collect from the bark of the trees, especially poplars, horse chestnut, spruce, larch, and other conifers (pine trees).

The bees coat the doorway of their hives with this substance and it stops any infection getting inside the hive. The bees also brush against it going in and out of the hive, thus protecting their home.

Propolis has been hospital-tested by numerous doctors over the years and it has been found to be effective against staphylococcus (throat-chest infections), salmonella (food poisoning) and E. coli (gastric infection).

External ulcers, such as leg ulcers, respond well to propolis, as do internal ulcers in the mouth, oesophagus, and stomach.

Propolis is particularly great for treating and warding off influenza.

There are no harmful side-effects, and best of all, propolis does not kill off the "good" bacteria in the gastrointestinal tract. It also boosts the immune system and helps to build up each person's resistance to infections (Note: in very rare cases, it has caused mild allergic reactions).

Garlic

Garlic is another well-known natural antibiotic that is particularly effective for fighting colds, coughs, and flu. It has natural antibiotic in it known as allicin and sulphur, long understood to be effective for bacterial infections.

Olive Leaf Extract

Another antibiotic alternative is olive leaf extract. Olive trees are among the world's oldest and longest living plants. The olive tree is particularly resistant to insects and microbial attraction. The olive leaves in particular concentrate large amounts of oleanolic acid. They act as a natural barrier to microbial invasion. Extracts of olive leaves have been used medicinally for several hundred years as it lowers fevers and treats malarial infections.

More recently, olive leaf extract has been shown to be a potent remedy against viral diseases, yeast and fungal infections, bacterial, protozoan, and parasite infections.

Colds, food poisoning, strep throat, warts, gastro, hepatitis, influenza, pneumonia, and ringworm, plus many other have all been successfully treated with olive leaf extract.

Echinacea

Echinacea is a herb well publicised for its terrific immune-building properties and its ability to handle upper-respiratory infections — coughs and the rhinovirus (common cold). It can shorten the duration of illness.

Grapefruit Seed Extract

Grapefruit seed extract is an excellent antibiotic, antifungal, and antiviral medicine. I discovered this medicine in America and I was so impressed with its effectiveness that we started a company (Citricidal Australia) to import it into Australia. We have received many letters from people who have successfully used grapefruit seed extract for various types of infections including fungal nails, Candida yeast infections, etc, especially those travelling to developing countries. People taking a small dose of "Traveler's Friend" (product name) just don't get diarrhoea.

Astragalus

There's also the Chinese herb Astragalus that is used extensively as a natural antibiotic and immune booster. Fantastic for flu and bacterial infections, we often use several of these together in our infections fighter.

Andrographis

This is an Ayurvedic medicine (Indian herbal medicine) which is also known to increase white cell count and assist your body to fight infections.

Goldenseal

Goldenseal is an English/European herbal medicine fantastic for staph infections and for colds, flu, and general inflammation. Goldenseal is great for catarrhal conditions such as chronic sinusitis.

The effects of antibiotics on the body

Medical antibiotics not only kill the "bad" or harmful bacteria but also destroy the "good" intestinal bacteria. This often causes deficiencies of vitamins B1 and B12 and can considerably lower a person's resistance to infection.

The destruction on the good intestinal bacteria is one of the major causes of the fungal infection Candida and vaginal thrush, which plagues so many women these days.

So if medical antibiotics are needed, ALWAYS take a strong probiotic (good bacteria) along with the prescribed medications. Take 1 hour away from such medications and at least 1 week after stopping the medical antibiotics.

I hope this information has been enlightening to you and alerts you to the fact we do have natural remedies for infections: remedies with all the benefits but without the harmful side-effects.

RESOURCE 7: Pregnancy Birthing Kit

1. Pulsatilla:	Strengthens contractions (take ½ hourly during 1st stage labour) and has been known to help turn breach babies: 10 drops 3x daily.
2. Caulophyllum:	(Blue Cohosh herb). Tones the uterus. 10 drops once daily, starting two weeks prior to due date. Also, during the first and second stages of labour if contractions become weaker or further apart. Helps regulate contractions: 10 drops ½ hourly to one hourly.
3. Arnica:	10 drops hourly during 2nd/3rd stage, then immediately after delivery of baby. Helps prevent hemorrhaging. If bleeding, take 10 drops every 10 minutes, until bleeding eases or stops, straight after birth. 10 drops 3x daily after delivery for two days – this helps swelling and bruising.
4. Rescue Remedy:	One of the Bach flower remedies made from flower essences. 10 drops as often as needed, up to every 10-15 minutes during 1st and 2nd stage of labour. Calms and settles emotions. Both mums and dads can benefit from this remedy. If the baby is very distressed, two drops on the tongue is very calming and soothing. Use every 10 minutes until baby has settled.

5. Kali Phos:	(Biochemic cell salt – Potassium Phosphate). Works as a nerve strengthener. Chew tablets or take drops up to every 15 minutes. Prevents exhaustion during labour and helps stop the shakes after delivery.
6. Vitamin C:	3000mg daily, from two weeks prior to due date. Helps strengthen wall of blood vessels, makes hemorrhaging less likely.
7. B Complex:	(Tresos B or Multi Essentials or Natal Care). Strengthens nerves prior to birth, for both mums and dads. One tablet morning and night, after food, two weeks prior to birth.
8. Raspberry Leaf:	Tea – one cup 3x daily or tonic – 5ml 3x daily. Aids delivery of placenta and tones uterus, thereby facilitating labour. Begin at 6th to 7th month of pregnancy. Also excellent in assisting the shrinking of uterus.
9. Colic Drops:	4 to 8 drops of Colic prior to feeding. For babies being bottle fed who suck in the air, silicon teats with side wings are recommended.

RESOURCE 8: Side-effects of the Contraceptive Pill

Hormones contained in the Pill can have side-effects which include increased risks of cervical, liver, and breast cancers, clots in legs, strokes, and heart attacks. Other potential side-effects include migraine, high blood pressure, food allergies, fluid retention, weight gain, thrush, depression, and increased risk of miscarriage and infertility.

Status of vital vitamins and minerals is altered by the Pill and affect women's health. Effects of the Pill on vitamins:

Vitamin A

Too much vitamin A is harmful to the human foetus. The Pill increases the circulating level of vitamin A; therefore stop taking the Pill three months before conceiving.

Vitamin B1

The Pill interferes with B1 metabolism and can cause a deficiency of vitamin B1.

Vitamin B2

Taking the Pill for long periods of time (three years or more) creates a B2 deficiency.

Vitamin B6

Taking the Pill alters the body's uptake of B6 and can lead to B6 deficiency, which can lead to fluid retention, impaired glucose tolerance, cancer of the urinary tract, dermatitis, and psychological problems (particularly depression).

Vitamin B12

An adverse effect of the Pill on vitamin B12 can lead to psychological disorders.

Folic Acid

The Pill interferes with blood cell formation by altering folic acid and B12 metabolism.

Vitamin C

Increased intake of vitamin C is needed when taking the Pill.

Vitamin E

The blood level of vitamin E decreases by 20% when a woman is on the Pill. Vitamin E is the fertility vitamin responsible for ovarian health.

Vitamin K

Taking the Pill increases levels of prothrombin, which means an increased likelihood of blood clots and can lead to chronic vascular disease, especially in smokers.

Effects of the Pill on minerals

Copper

As in pregnancy, women on the Pill have increased levels of serum copper.

Zinc

Increased serum copper causes low plasma zinc.

Iron

Women on the Pill can have low iron levels (Anaemia). Excess tea and coffee intake also causes iron loss.

Which Doctor?

Magnesium

It is common for women on the Pill to be deficient in magnesium.

Recommended nutritional supplementation

(For women coming off the Pill or if the Pill causes you to feel unwell)

- B complex, including Folic Acid
- Vitamin C, 2000mg per day
- Vitamin E, 500 IU per day
- Magnesium, 200mg per day
- Zinc, 25mg per day (with manganese)
- Amino acid supplements for aided fat metabolism

Please note: All nutritional supplement recommendations should be adjusted by your practitioner to suit individual needs. A healthy diet is also highly recommended.

RESOURCE 9: The Most Pervasive Form of Child Abuse

The woman's hand closes around the baby's throat. Then she presses, slowly strangling the baby. The defenceless infant struggles. Just in time, the woman relaxes her grip. The baby gasps for air but survives the assault. Before long the woman grabs the tiny throat again, starting the torture all over. Again, she lets go and leaves the infant gasping.

What you just read describes the suffering experienced by an unborn child when abused by its smoking mother.

Lifelong Damage

An overstatement? Hardly. A *New York Times* article reports that increasing numbers of scientific studies show that a mother who smokes regularly may impose lifelong physical and mental handicaps upon her child. Some of these injuries, says the article, "Are immediately apparent while others develop more slowly".

In what way does a mother's smoking affect the unborn child? Dr William G Cahan, an attending surgeon at the Memorial Sloan Kettering Cancer Centre in the United States and author of the *Times* article, explains: "Within minutes, each cigarette puff introduces carbon monoxide and nicotine into the maternal blood."

As the carbon monoxide reduces the blood's ability to carry oxygen and the nicotine constricts the blood vessels in the placenta, "the unborn child is temporarily deprived of its normal amount of oxygen. If this deprivation is repeated often enough," says surgeon Cahan, "it could irreparably damage the fetal brain, an organ uniquely sensitive to a lack of oxygen."

One study, for instance, revealed that five minutes after pregnant women smoked only two cigarettes, their fetuses showed signs of distress – accelerated heart rate accompanied by abnormal breathing like movements.

Pack-a-day Smokers

What, then, are the implications for an unborn child if its mother smokes 20 cigarettes, or one pack, a day? Dr Cahan figures that an average smoker inhales five puffs per cigarette. Thus, a pack a day habit amounts to a hundred puffs a day. With pregnancy lasting about 270 days, the mother subjects the fetus "to at least 27,000 physical chemical insults."

Such abused babies may pay a lifelong price for their mother's tobacco habit. Besides physical problems, says Dr Cahan, the children may have "behavioral problems, impaired reading abilities, hyperactivity, and mental retardation." Not surprisingly, he asks: "What responsible woman can persist in a habit so threatening to her young?"

In addition, smoking parents are also a threat to growing children. Why? The booklet *Facts & Figures on Smoking*, published by the American Cancer Society, answers "children of smokers have more respiratory illnesses than those of nonsmokers, including an increase in the frequency of bronchitis and pneumonia in early life." Dr Cahan therefore concludes that, "this form of child abuse may be the most pervasive of all." The question is, do you choose to avoid it?

RESOURCE 10: Preconception care

1. To provide your body with the 'building blocks' necessary to create a healthy baby, you need to eat healthy and nutritious whole foods. This means buying fresh, unrefined foods that have been fed or grown organically and therefore have a plentiful supply of nutrients.

2. To avoid the toxins that come through your water and food supply, such as agrochemicals and heavy metals, you need to use a water purifier and buy organic foods whenever possible. This is especially important with animal products, in which the animals may have been fed hormones or antibiotics, or have been exposed to polluting chemicals, as these collect in the fatty tissue and organs of the animals.

3. Avoid sugar (and all sugar substitutes), coffee (also decaffeinated), and alcohol as these contribute to nutrient loss. Eat plenty of vegetables (raw and cooked), whole grains and protein-providing foods, but avoid saturated fats (animal and heated). Avoid all chemical additives and highly processed foods. Read your labels carefully and buy fresh produce whenever possible.

4. Drink dandelion tea (or coffee) – which is an excellent detoxifying herb through its action on the liver – and eat plenty of garlic which also helps to eliminate toxins. Better still, consult a medical herbalist for a holistic approach to detoxification and reproductive health.

5. To avoid chemical oestrogen mimics in the environment, which can contribute to reproductive disease and fertility problems in both sexes, you should, again, eat organically fed animal produce and avoid keeping or heating foods in plastic wrap. To protect the

nutritional content of your food, you should also avoid using pre-prepared and packaged foods or foods that have been microwaved.

6. Take a comprehensive nutrient supplement, including the complete range of vitamins, minerals, and essential fatty acids. These are required for proper fertility and healthy embryonic growth. The antioxidant nutrients, vitamin A, C, and E, zinc, and selenium, can help you to detoxify and eliminate heavy metals and chemicals. A hair analysis can give you information on nutrient status and heavy metal residue in your body.

7. Avoid all drugs. This includes social drugs such as alcohol, caffeine, and nicotine, all of which have been linked to reproductive and foetal ill health. Also avoid medicinal drugs except if they are medically prescribed and where they cannot be safely replaced with a natural alternative.

8. Avoid breathing in petrol fumes or using household cleaning materials which are ammonia-based or any solvents. Studies have shown that oven cleaners, mould treatments, paint, glues, and all solvents can affect the health of sperm or eggs. Now is not the time to renovate your house or have it treated for pests.

9. Have a thorough and comprehensive screening for genitourinary infections in both partners.

10. To avoid the effects of non-ionising radiation, use your mobile phone and microwave as little as possible, and keep it away from your body. Further exposure comes from computer screens. Turn the monitor off when not in use, hang an anti-radiation screen in front of it, and place a cushion stuffed with Epsom salts on your lap. These absorb radiation, and, as they do so, the crystals will break down into a powder when they need to be replaced.

11. To avoid the most toxic, ionizing form of radiation, which can affect eggs and sperm for up to three years, avoid X-rays for as long as possible before conception, and only fly if really unavoidable, as one flight exposes you to the equivalent of a full body X-ray.

12. Exercise for at least two hours per week, and try to normalise your weight. This should be made easier by eating healthy foods.

13. For stress, which can be a problem for those who've been trying to conceive for a while, an effective remedy is to lie down in a quiet place, with no interruptions, and direct breath to each part of your body in turn. Then you can create pictures in your head of the positive outcome of an easy conception, successful pregnancy and birthing, and a beautiful, healthy baby. If stress is an ongoing problem, it can affect your nutritional status and fertility, so if this simple self-help remedy does not fully address the issue, seek other forms of stress relief/management or professional help.

All of these measures should be in place for at least four months before conception, as this is how long it takes for sperm to generate and eggs to mature, during which time they are vulnerable to toxicity and nutrient deficiencies.

RESOURCE 11: Diet Post Menopause

Principles Include

A. Utilising plant sources of phytoestrogens.

B. Increasing calcium intake.

C. Increasing fibre intake.

D. A lower total calorie intake.

A. Phytoestrogens

Soy foods (tofu, tempeh, soy milk)

Red kidney beans, pinto beans, chickpeas, and split peas

Linseeds, almonds, sunflower seeds, sesame seeds

Alfalfa sprouts, soy sprouts, mung bean sprouts

B. Total calcium intake of 1200 – 1500 mg daily

This may be obtained from foods or with supplements as a back-up to dietary intake.

Calcium citrate and calcium phosphate are preferable forms of calcium for assimilation. The inclusion of magnesium, silicon, and boron is an added benefit for improved assimilation and ultimate bone strength.

Calcium-rich foods include:

Salmon	Cabbage
Broccoli	Hazelnuts
Sardines	Spinach
Parsley	Sunflower seeds
Almonds	Yoghurt
Figs	Pumpkin seeds
Rolled oats	Cottage cheese

C. High Fibre Diet:

This is beneficial in terms of reducing cholesterol levels. It is also a useful long-term preventative for bowel cancer.

A delicious mixture of grains which is both calcium rich and phytoestrogen rich as well as high in fibre is the seed mix:

Linseeds

Oat bran	equal parts grind/ blend
Almonds	to a suitable consistency
Sesame seeds	2 dessert spoons daily

Sunflower seeds

Pumpkins seeds

Seed mix can be added to cereal, yoghurt, stewed fruits, or even salad. It is very tasty.

Plants Sources of Oestrogens:

Phytoestrogenic foods may be included in the diet as part of the natural therapies management of menopausal and postmenopausal symptoms.

Which Doctor?

1. Legumes:

- Including soy foods (such as soy milk, tofu, tempeh)
- Red kidney beans, pinto beans, chickpeas, split peas, and lentils
- French beans (1 serving is 1 cup)

2. Nuts and seeds:

- Linseeds
- Almonds
- Sunflowers seeds
- Pumpkin seeds (1 serving is ½ cup)

3. Sprouts:

- Alfalfa spouts
- Red clover sprouts
- Soy bean sprouts
- Fenugreek sprouts (1 serving is 1 cup)

Consuming 1 serving of phytoestrogen rich foods 5 days a week is sufficient to benefit from their effects.

Phytoestrogens have an oestrogenic action in women whose oestrogen levels are low.

Phytoestrogens can be beneficial in minimising menopausal symptoms such as hot flushes, dry skin, urinary frequency, and vaginal soreness.

They are considered to be safe for use by women who have a history of breast cancer and there is evidence that they can be useful preventatives for this condition when used long term as part of the diet. It is the oestradiol, the synthetic oestrogen that is potentially carcinogenic, not the phytoestrogens.

RESOURCE 12: Birth Plan

Contact Details:

Mother:

Father:

Support person:

- We ask that our birth intentions be honoured as medically possible. Our decisions are based on personal research and education. Rest assured that we will cooperate with you in any medical emergency and are open to all suggestions if medically needed for Mother or the baby.

- We plan to have a drug-free birth. We are aware of our pain relief options and will request them if wanted. Please do not suggest any drug pain relief unless requested.

- We request that the birth environment be kept as silent and natural as medically possible. We would like the lights to be kept dim during the birth and talking and noise to a minimum as medically possible during labour.

- We would like to use the bath and shower once labour is established.

- We will be using homeopathic drops before, during, and after the birth for both Mother and Father as needed.

- We request no internal vaginal exams unless you feel it is absolutely medically necessary.

- We request not to have the Mother's membranes ruptured unless medically indicated.

- We request that labour be allowed to progress in the most natural way possible with as little intervention as possible unless there is a medical indication or emergency.

- We ask that a caesarean be used as a last resort unless the life of the baby or Mother is in immediate danger.

- We would prefer to risk a tear rather than an episiotomy, unless the baby is distressed and needs to be born immediately.

- If the birth is straightforward and no intervention is required, we would like a physiological third stage.

- We would like immediate skin-to-skin contact by the baby being placed on Mother's stomach with the cord to be clamped only after pulsation have stopped and then cut by the Father.

- We intend to breastfeed and request that the baby be offered the breast as soon as possible and that the baby not be removed from Mother for as long as possible unless for some medical reason.

- We request that **no** formula be given to the baby unless medically needed.

- We request that weighing and measuring of the baby be held off as long as possible for maximum bonding time with parents, and that when it does happen, for it be done in the presence of Mother or Father.

- We ask that Father accompany the baby at all times when away from Mother and that no medical procedures be performed on the baby, including vaccination, without our consent.

- If labour is straightforward and the baby does not have any cuts or minimal bruising, we ask that no vitamin K be given to the baby.

If you feel it is medically needed, we ask that it be discussed with us first.

- We request that no hepatitis B vaccines are given to the baby.
- We request that no vaccines are given to Mother or baby without prior consent.
- We would prefer to bathe the baby the day after birth.
- Please discuss with us, time permitting, why and what intervention may be required and allow us to be involved in the decision. You will have our full cooperation if medical intervention is needed for our baby's safety.

In absence of complication, we ask that our requests be honoured. Thank you for your support and cooperation.

Mother:

Father:

RESOURCE 13: Weight Loss Plan

Chinese Herbal Medicine has been practised for thousands of years with great emphasis being placed on extensive and continuous research into the treatment of disease and promotion of good health.

There are four main components to this programme:

1. Herbal Medicine Chinese Herbs
2. Guidelines for a sensible eating plan
3. A routine of moderate exercise
4. A level of commitment

Being the correct weight for your height is one of the components that makes for a healthy mind and body; builds self-esteem and confidence; makes you look and feel great.

With a program of herbal medicine, healthy diet, and moderate exercise, we can help you achieve the body you want.

On this diet, you can expect to lose at least two kilograms per week.

The medicinal herbs integral to this program have several important functions. It must be stressed, however, that the herbs alone or the diet plan alone will not achieve the expected results. The two components must work together in order to operate at peak efficiency.

The herbs can be roughly divided into four categories according to function:

* To promote natural and gentle diuretic action

* To assist the metabolism in the fat conversion process

* A powerful yet gentle stimulant for liver activity to aid in the detoxification process
* Herbs to enable the body to absorb more the nutrients available in the food being eaten

Instructions:

Multivitamin and mineral capsule (if indicated, one capsule daily in the morning.)

Herbal medicine, 3 capsules x2 daily – Chinese Weight Loss Herbs.

The Eating Plan:

Day 1:

Eat all the fruit you want all day, especially melons (no bananas)

Soup, all you want.

Day 2:

All the vegetables you want, freshly cooked or raw, including salad (except peas, corn, beans, potatoes, and lentils)

Or 50g fish

Or 1 poached/boiled egg

Or 50g skinned lean chicken or beef

Soup anytime, all you want.

Day 3:

All fruits and vegetables, including salad (no bananas)

Soup anytime, all you want

1 baked potato with butter from the daily allowance.

Day 4:

All vegetables, including salad

100g of tofu/bean curd

Or 100g fish

Or 2 poached/boiled eggs

Or 4oz (110g) skinned lean chicken

Soup anytime

1 banana.

Day 5:

All fruits (no bananas) and vegetables, including salads (no potatoes, peas, corn, dried beans, lentils)

Soup anytime, all you want.

Day 6:

All vegetables, including salad

Or 50g fish

Or 1 poached/boiled egg

Or 50g skinned lean chicken or 50g lean beef

Soup anytime, all you want.

Day 7:

Brown organic rice, fruit and vegetables, all you can eat

Soup anytime, all you want.

Please avoid the use of pumpkins and any other root vegetables: these contain a high amount of starch. The exceptions are potatoes when they are indicated on the eating plan; beetroot, if raw (eg if grated on salad); and carrot, cooked or raw.

Soup:

3 medium onions, leek or spring onion

1 – 2 sticks of celery

6 button mushrooms

¼ cabbage

1 zucchini

400g fresh tomatoes or 1 tin peeled tomatoes (sugar free)

1 green pepper

1 vegetable stock cube (MSG free) eg Massel / bone broth

Cut up vegetables, place in a large saucepan. Cover with water.

Boil for 10 minutes. Cover and simmer over a low heat until vegetables are soft.

Other vegetables can be added according to taste. However, avoid vegetables that contain high amounts of carbohydrates, such as potatoes.

Daily Allowances:

300ml skim milk, soy milk, rice or oat milk, almond milk, preferably vegetable oil free.

25g butter

x2 crispbread or plain crackers or x3 rice cakes or x2 flat mountain bread (wheat free).

Please note:

All meat or fish must be grilled, baked, or poached without oil.

Which Doctor?

Meat should also be lean and trimmed of fat and skin.

Eggs should be poached or boiled.

As much water as desired.

Green or herbal tea is acceptable.

Note: This diet is not suitable for diabetics.

RESOURCE 14: Anti Cancer Foods

BROCCOLI SPROUTS

The cruciferous vegetables, eg broccoli, cabbage, cauliflower, and brussel sprouts, contain substances called isothiocyanates, which are potent activators of enzymes in the body which inactivate carcinogens, and hence protect against cancer. Broccoli and cauliflower are rich in the isothiocyanate glucoraphanin, but 3-day old sprouts from the seeds contain 10 to 100 times as much as the mature vegetable.

Rats who were fed extracts of 3-day old sprouts developed fewer and less rapidly growing mammary tumours induced by chemical carcinogens than the rats who were not fed the extracts.

Hence, eating broccoli sprouts may be as useful for humans in protecting against the risk of cancer.

Ref: Fahey J.W. et al – Proc, Nat. Acad. Sciences- 1997;94: 10367-10372

RASPBERRIES AND POMEGRANATES

Certain fruits contain ellagic acid, a proven inducer of apoptosis: the process by which normal, non-malignant cells exhibit a self-limited lifespan. Cancer cells grow out of control without the normal processes of limitation because the cell apoptosis mechanisms have been switched off.

Ellagic acid content of foods: mcg/mg

Pomegranate – 15,200

Raspberries – 1,460

Figs – 517

Strawberries – also quite rich, but if not organic, they may be toxic with pesticides.

Raspberry puree fed to experimental animals with cancer has been shown to shrink tumours. Raspberries are currently being tested in long-term clinical trials in the USA in cancer patients and in healthy subjects (prospective studies). These trials may confirm a suspected cancer-inhibiting effect of raspberries by virtue of its content of ellagic acid.

Source: Dr Daniel Nixon – Gawler Foundation Conference, 8 August 1998

Pomegranates are in season March to April in Victoria. Organic pomegranate juice is available from Health Food Shops ('Lakewood', about $20 and 'Found', $14) and is a good fruit juice to have with the large oral doses of vitamin C recommended for cancer patients. Cheaper pomegranate juices, eg 'Desert Dunes' from Cedar Bakery, 33 High St. Preston, may also be OK.

TURMERIC

Turmeric contains curcumin which has several cancer-retarding properties. Curcumin:

Suppresses the nuclear growth factor kappa beta (NF-KB) which tends to fuel malignant cell proliferation and inhibit cell growth at the G2 stage.

Blocks cancer by promoting chemicals such as xenoestrogens and nitrosamines.

Protects against oxidative damage to cell DNA, eg by radiation.

Helps to normalise the deficient cell apoptosis (self-destruction) mechanisms of malignant cells.

Inhibits angiogenesis necessary for tumour growth.

Enhances cell immunity.

Absorption of curcumin is enhanced by piperine added to capsules of curcumin.

GREEN TEA

This is best as powder mixed with carrot juice and is recommended to cancer patients: boiling water destroys the catechins in green tea. Green tea catechins induce tumour cell apoptosis and have other beneficial functions that may assist in retarding cancer cell proliferation and disease progression.

TOMATOES contain lycopene, an antioxidant that may retard some cancers by inhibiting the stimulatory effects of IGF-1 on cancer cell proliferation.

ONIONS contain quercetin, an antioxidant that induces apoptosis and may retard many cancers.

GARLIC contains allicin, which may retard some cancers by inducing apoptosis, inhibiting proliferation, and stimulating NK cell activity against cancer cells.

The bioavailability of these is enhanced by lightly cooking in cold-pressed extra virgin olive oil.

RESOURCE 15: Acid Alkaline Foods

According to scientific research, it has been definitely determined that a body should be nearly as alkaline as possible. However, to have a perfectly alkaline body would be impossible as well as incorrect. When one speaks of an acidic body, it means that the body is no longer near the alkaline point. Most disease begins with acidity in the system, causing inflammation, pain, and many other unnatural symptoms.

The following table is a list of acid and alkaline foods which, if consumed correctly, can cure many of the problems of health we are faced with today. Correct food combinations are essential for proper and efficient digestion and assimilation.

The suggested ration for good health and fast recovery is 80% alkaline and 20% healthy acid foods, 5% to 10% more acids may be taken in very cold climates, as these are also heat and energy sources.

Do well and you will reap the rewards.

ALKALINE

Fruits

Apples/Cider

Apricots

Avocados

Bananas (Speckled)

Berries

Cantaloupe

Carob (pod)

Cranberries

Cherries

Currents

Dates

Figs

Grapes

Grapefruit

Kumquats

Lemons (Ripe)

Limes

Mangoes

Melons

Nectarines

Olives (Sun Dried)

Oranges

Papayas (Paw Paw)

Passionfruit

Peaches

Pears

Pineapple (fresh)

Plums

Pomegranates

Prunes

Quinces

Raisins

Tamarind

Tomatoes

Vegetables

Asparagus (Ripe)

Bamboo Shoots

Beans (Green, Lima, Spouts, String)

Broccoli

Cabbage (Red & White)

Carrots

Celery

Cauliflower

Chard

Chicory

Chives

Collard

Cowslip Cucumber

Dandelion Greens

Dill

Dock

Dulse (Sea Lettuce)

Eggplant

Endives

Garlic

Horse Radish (fresh)

Jerusalem Artichoke

Kale

Kohlrabi

Leeks

Legumes (Except Peanuts and Lentils)

Lettuce

Mushrooms Onions

Parsley

Parsnips

Peppers (Green & Red)

Potatoes

Pumpkin

Radish

Sauerkraut

Sorrel

Soya Bean & Extracts

Spinach

Squash

Turnips

Water Chestnuts

Watercress

Dairy Products

Acidophilus

Buttermilk

Milk (raw, human, cow or goat only if unprocessed or unheated)

Whey Yoghurt

Flesh Foods

None. Blood & Bone only are alkaline forming.

Cereals

Corn (Green)

Millet

Buckwheat

Nuts

Almonds (Raw)

Chestnuts (Roasted)

Coconut (Raw)

Cashews (Raw)

Miscellaneous

Agar

Alfalfa Products

Coffee Substitute

Ginger (Unsweetened)

Honey

Kelp

Teas (Unsweetened)

ACID

Fruits

All preserved, canned, jellied, sugared, glazed or sulphured fruits. Bananas with green tips

Olives (Pickled and Green)

Rhubarb

Vegetables

Artichokes

Asparagus tips

Benan (All Dried)

Brussels Sprouts

Lentils

Dairy Product

Butter

Cheese

Cottage Cheese

Cream, Ice Cream, Ices

Custard

Milk (Boiled, Cooked, Malted, Pasteurised, Dried & Canned)

Flesh Foods

All Meat, Fowl & Fish

Beef Tea (Bonox)

Gelatin

Gravies

Cereals

All Flour Products

Barley

Bread of all Kinds

Cakes

Corn, Corn Meal,
Cornflakes

Doughnuts

Dumplings

Macaroni/Spaghetti

Noodles

Oatmeal

Pies & Pastries

Rice

Rye Biscuits

Miscellaneous

All Alcoholic
Beverages

Candy &
Confectionery Cocoa

Chocolate

Coca Cola

Coffee

Condiments such as
Curry, Salt, Pepper &
Spices

Drugs of all kinds
incl. Aspirin

Eggs (esp. the whites)

Ginger (Preserved)

Jams & Jellies

Flavorings

Marmalades

Preservatives

Sago

Salt

Soda Water

Tapioca

Tobacco

Vinegar

Lack of Sleep Worry

Stress

Overwork

Neutral

Sugar (Refined)

Oils (Olive, Corn,
Peanut, Soy, Sesame)

Brown Rice

NOTE: Sugars yield
an alkaline ash (if
burned) but its effect
on the blood stream
in high concentration
is highly acidic.
Whilst fruit is acid
outside the body,
after digestion and
absorption has
occurred it has an
alkaline effect on the
blood stream.

*List taken from the work
of Rex Lloyd, Health
Research, California,
USA*

RESOURCE 16: Laser Therapy

What is Cold Laser Therapy?

Cold Laser Therapy is a non-invasive drug-free option that offers a natural solution to pain management. The cold laser device emits 4 radiances of light that identify and target inflamed tissue without damaging healthy tissue. The different lasers have been proven to quickly and effectively reduce inflammation, giving the body the best environment to heal and relieve pain. It can be used alone or in combination with other natural therapies. It is ideal for those who wish to avoid surgery or drugs.

What does it treat?	Benefits of Cold Laser Therapy
Cold Laser Therapy can effectively resolve chronic and acute pain in many conditions including: • Bursitis • Back pain • Carpal tunnel • Arthritis pain • Tennis elbow • Fibromyalgia • Muscle strain • Tendonitis • Soft tissue injuries • Many other conditions	• Non-Toxic • Non-Invasive • Very little or no contra-indications • Easy to apply • Very Safe • Cost Effective • Highly effective for the patient • No side-effects or pain • Alternative to analgesics, NSAIDs and other medications.

How many sessions are required?

A result may be noticed after the first treatment, however for optimum results 3-10 sessions are usually recommended depending on the duration and severity of the condition.

RESOURCE 17: The Cleansing Response

Detoxification

Over time, our bodies accumulate toxins – from pesticides and other chemicals in processed foods, from impure air and water, from medications, from poor digestions and elimination, etc.

Whenever the metabolism isn't able to remove a toxic molecule, it must store it in the body, typically in the liver or fatty tissues. Later, when the metabolism is stronger because of better nutrition, exercise, improved hormone balance, reduced stress, etc, it will start to flush out the toxins. This "cleansing process" is part of the body's natural health building process.

Cleansing Reactions

For some people, however, the process of eliminating the stored toxins is uncomfortable enough to warrant attention. These are often the people who can gain the most from taking steps to rebuild their health. It often happens that someone who feels worse after starting a nutritional program feels *much* better after the initial cleansing reaction is completed.

Fatigue, headache, flu-like symptoms, skin reactions, mood changes, changing sleep patterns, digestive reactions, aches and pains, allergic symptoms, etc, may occur or increase during the cleansing process.

What type of reaction occurs depends on the unique body chemistry and state of health of each individual. While most people notice no reaction at all, some do experience one or more of those listed – or some other reaction according to their body's own functioning.

What to do

These suggestions are good for *everyone*, regardless of whether you're experiencing any discomfort.

1. Drink plenty of water (purified, if possible) every day. One litre per 45 kilograms of body weight is a good rule of thumb. This helps flush the toxins from the cells, and it help the kidneys with their natural cleansing function.

2. Include fibre-containing foods in your diet, especially fresh vegetables and whole fresh fruits. You may choose to use a dietary fibre product containing psyllium or other bulk-forming fibre sources. The fibre helps absorb toxins and "sweep out" the digestive tract.

3. Try to eat mainly fresh, whole foods. Avoid processed foods, refined foods, and foods containing toxins and "anti-nutrients" (sugars, caffeine, alcohol, artificial flavours and colours, chemicals, etc). This will reduce the work of processing unhealthy foods, and it increases the available nutrition for your body to rebuild itself.

4. Reduce your exposure to environmental toxins and pollutants. Allow fresh air in your living and working places; avoid fumes from strong-smelling products; reduce your exposure to cigarette smoke, etc. Reducing your daily load makes it easier for your body to get rid of toxins.

5. Exercise. Pick an amount and type of exercise that is right for your state of health (check with your doctor if you have any doubts). For most people, walking at least 15 minutes a day is a good way to start. Exercise increases circulation, respiration, and cellular metabolism. It helps the body burn off toxins and wastes and/or pump them out of the system.

6. Listen to your body and do whatever you need to stay within a manageable comfort zone. You may find that a smaller helping of a particular nutritional product is better for you, either temporarily while there is a strong cleansing response, or long term due to your individual body chemistry. You may even decide that a particular supplement simply isn't right for you.

If a cleansing reaction is too strong, you can reduce or even stop taking supplements for a few days until you feel better, then gradually build back up to a regular daily amount. (Some people need to go very slowly, using very small amounts for a while. These are often the people who eventually have the most dramatic transformation in wellbeing if they follow through.) You may need to repeat this cycle more than once.

7. If a symptom causes concern, check with a health professional. Some symptoms may be unrelated to the body's response or the healing response itself may draw attention to an underlying problem.

RESOURCE 18: MTHFR Gene Mutation

MTHFR specifically is a gene that holds the recipe (instructions) for the enzyme methylenetetrahydrofolate reductase. When functioning properly, it is highly efficient at helping our bodies convert vitamin B9 (folate), folic acid, into a usable form called methylfolate. This process is called methylation.

When the MTHFR gene is mutated, the capacity to convert vitamin B9 into methylfolate is reduced by 40% to 70%. Converting folate into a usable form is essential for DNA (protein building blocks) synthesis and repair, neurotransmitter production, eg serotonin, melatonin, dopamine (just to name a few), detoxification, and immune function.

In simpler terms, imagine your DNA is a cookbook and your genes that give instructions to your cells are the recipes within that cookbook. If one of those recipes got a little mixed up (gene mutation), it can affect all the other recipes within that cookbook that call for that same recipe (gene).

Essentially that is what a mutation is – a slight change to the instructions that can have sometimes small, sometimes significant, impacts on other genes.

The "folate in most processed fortified foods like cereals and bakery goods and vitamins is folic acid which is harmful to those with the gene mutation."

Are all MTHFR mutations the same?

No. There are over 50 types of MTHFR gene mutations, possibly more that have yet to be discovered. The two that are most commonly studied and tested for are C677T and A1298C.

C677T mutation

- We inherit one copy of each gene from our mother and father. If you test positive for the C677T mutation, there are two possibilities.
- Heterozygous – having one copy of the C677T mutation and one normal copy translating to an estimated 40% loss of function.
- Homozygous – having two copies of the C677T mutation translating to an estimated 70% loss of function.

A1298C mutation

- There is debate about whether those with the A1298C mutation experience diminished function. Some say no, but in our experience, we definitely witness it!

In cases where an individual is compound heterozygous – having one C677T mutation and one A1298C mutation – there is an estimated 50% loss of function.

What could MTHFR gene mutation affect?

Researchers have found a connection between MTHFR gene mutation and tongue and lip ties, heart disease, Alzheimer's, recurrent miscarriage, asthma, prostate cancer, bladder cancer, multiple sclerosis type symptoms, anxiety, depression, insomnia, and severe PMT.

Can we supplement with folic acid?

Unfortunately, folic acid – which is a synthetic vitamin found in fortified foods and almost all vitamin supplements – is considered harmful to people with MTHFR mutations. People who have low levels of the MTHFR enzyme are not able to convert it into a usable form. The unconverted folic acid attaches itself to the same receptors in the body used to absorb folate, effectively blocking the body's ability to absorb any usable folate consumed from your green vegetables.

Note: Many lab tests do not distinguish between folic acid and folate when measuring blood levels. If folic acid intake is high, the results may show an individual has adequate amounts of folate when, in fact, what they actually have are high levels of unusable folic acid but very little of the natural folate.

The good news!

Our DNA is not our destiny. It is like a musical instrument. In order to make music, it needs something – or someone – to play it. That something is epigenetics, which means "above" genetics. The epigenome is a second genome that plays like the first violin in the orchestra, turning genes on and off according to the sheet music.

That sheet music is our lifestyle: the food we eat; how we interact with stress; whether or not we get enough sleep; and for those with the MTHFR mutation, how you compensate for it in order to support overall function.

You have the MTHFR mutation. What now?

Unfortunately, there is no one-size-fits-all approach to MTHFR. Supplementation with methylfolate (labelled as 5 L-MTHF or 6(S)-L-MTHF) is often recommended along with vitamin B12 in the form of SL methylcobalamin or hydroxocobalamin.

However, there are cases in which supplementation can cause serious side-effects, especially when high doses are introduced at the beginning. This is often the case when the individual has other genetic mutations that interact with MTHFR or especially toxic buildup that can cause severe detox reactions when one's liver cannot cope with methylating out these toxins, hence the experience of brain fog.

It is recommended that you consult with an experienced healthcare practitioner with good knowledge of MTHFR Gene Mutation.

How to get tested for MTHFR

Your natural healthcare practitioner or your GP can refer you to a specialist laboratory. Children can also be affected and should be tested also.

RESOURCE 19: Pyrrole Disorder

What is Pyrrole Disorder?

Pyrrole disorder, also known as pyroluria, kryptopyrroluria, kryptopyrrole, or Mauve disorder can be inherited genetically or acquired through environmental and emotional stress, especially from 'leaky gut syndrome' and the overuse of antibiotics.

It can be best described as an abnormality in the production of haemoglobin that causes an overproduction of a by product called **hydroxyhempyrolin** (HPL). The HPL binds to zinc and B6, starving the body of those nutrients causing a variety of symptoms. HPL is also a biomarker for oxidative stress and is neurotoxic. Stress of any kind will increase production of pyrroles/HPL which, in turn, decreases levels of zinc and B6 in the body.

Signs and Symptoms

The main characteristics manifest as severe zinc and B6 deficiency. Zinc is essential for healing, immune function, digestion, neurotransmitter activation, physical growth, memory, insulin sensitivity, control of blood sugars, DNA replication, and many more other functions.

Things to watch out for:

- White spots on fingernails is a strong sign of this zinc deficiency problem.
- Hypoglycemia/sugar intolerance is common, as are food and environmental allergies.

- Joint pains (especially knee pain).
- Fatigue.
- Headaches, migraines, and sensitivity to light.
- Bowel dysfunction, such as irritable bowel syndrome.
- Bruising easily.
- Dizziness, insomnia, poor memory, and difficulty concentrating.
- Learning difficulties such as ADHD.
- Stress, anxiety, panic attacks, mood swings, poor short-term memory, and depression.

Conditions associated with Pyroluria

A study led by orthomolecular psychiatrist Abram Hoffer found that pyroluria was frequently present in people with the following conditions:

- Acute intermittent porphyria 100%.
- Latent acute intermittent porphyria 70%.
- Down's syndrome 71%.
- Schizophrenia, acute 59 – 80%.
- Schizophrenia, chronic 40 – 50%.
- Criminal behaviour in adults, sudden deviance 71%.
- Criminal behaviour in youths, violent offenders 33%.
- Manic depression 47 – 50%.
- Depression, non-schizophrenic 12 – 46%.
- Autism 46 – 48%. (Including Asperger's Syndrome, Tourette's Syndrome).
- Epilepsy 44%.

- Learning difficulties and disability / ADHD / ADD 40 – 47%.

- Neuroses, neurotic behaviour 20%.

- Alcoholism 20 – 84%.

Diagnosis

Most people with pyroluria suffer from some of the symptoms above. A more definitive diagnosis can be made with a urine test.

Treatment

Pyroluria is managed in part by restoring vitamin B6 and zinc. This type of replacement therapy is very important as zinc must be provided in an efficiently absorbed form. Vitamin B6 is also available in several forms. Other nutrients that may assist include niacinamide (B3), pantothenic acid (B5), methylcobalamin (B12), manganese, vitamins C, E, and magnesium.

In mild cases, improvement can be seen in a couple of days. With more severe cases, it may take between 3 and 6 months to abate. If treatment stops, symptoms can return within a couple of days.

RESOURCE 20: Biogenetic Hair analysis

Is your body nutritionally balanced? Do you know if your environment is having an effect on your wellness? Could toxins and pathogens be affecting you negatively?

Now, for the first time ever, you can find out these answers and more and have your own personally optimised wellness plan generated – all in less than 15 minutes. How do we do it? Via a simple in-house Bio Genetic Hair Follicle Analysis. With only 4 strands of hair including your follicles, we can assess your health! This technology scans your hair, the information is then emailed to Cell Wellbeing in Germany and your 30-page report is generated.

There are many daily environmental factors which can affect the way in which our genes express themselves and therefore influence our cellular strengths or weaknesses. How your personal environment impacts your health, will be highlighted for you! Using our revolutionary German Bio-feedback technology, we are able to return a complete Environmental Wellness Report to your in less than 15 minutes, directly from Germany. This wellness report will highlight areas of cellular weakness, such as:

- Toxins - chemicals, metals, pesticides
- Microbiology - bacteria, fungus, parasites, virus
- Diet - food sensitivities
- Electromagnetic Fields & Radiation (wi-fi, mobiles)
- Vitamins & minerals
- Omega 3, 6, 9 oils

- Antioxidants
- Amino acids

This can all be done by post.

For more information, contact our Ferny Creek Clinic on 03 9755 1900

www.naturalhealingcentre.com.au

RESOURCE 21: Liver and Gallbladder

Cleansing the liver and gallbladder has everything to do with gaining your health back. It dramatically improves digestion, which is the basis of your whole health. You can expect your allergies to disappear too, more with each cleanse you do! Incredibly, it also eliminates shoulder, upper arm, and upper back pain. You have more energy and an increased sense of wellbeing.

It is the job of the liver to make bile, 1 to 1 ½ quarts in a day! The liver is full of tubes (biliary tubing) that delivers the bile to one large tube (common bile duct). The gallbladder is attached to the common bile duct and acts as a storage reservoir. Eating fat or protein triggers the gallbladder to squeeze itself after about 20 minutes, then the stored bile finishes its trip down the common bile duct to the intestine. There are other substances that can trigger the gallbladder, such as red pepper (cayenne), ginger, and fruit acids. Note: fruit juice is the first thing you have after a cleanse.

Cleansing the liver bile ducts is the most powerful procedure that you can do to improve your body's health, but it should not be done before the parasite program.

For best results, follow the kidney cleanse and any dental work you need.

For many people, including children, the biliary tubing in the liver is choked with gallstones. Some develop allergies or hives but some have no symptoms. When the gallbladder is scanned or X-rayed, nothing is seen. Typically, they are not in the gallbladder. Not only that, most are too small and not calcified, a prerequisite for visibility on X-ray.

There are over half a dozen varieties of gallstones, most of which have cholesterol crystals in them. They can be black, red, white, or tan coloured. The green ones get their colour from being coated with bile. At the very centre of each stone is a clump of bacteria, suggesting a dead bit of parasite might have started the stone forming. As the stones grow and become more numerous, the back pressure on the liver causes it to make less bile. Imagine the situation if your garden hose had marbles in it: much less water would flow, which, in turn, would decrease the ability of the hose to squirt out the marbles. With gallstones, much less cholesterol leaves the body, and cholesterol levels may rise.

Gallstones, being porous, can pick up all bacteria, cysts, viruses, and parasites that are passing through the liver. In this way, "nests" of infection are formed, forever supplying the body with fresh bacteria. No stomach infection such as ulcers or intestinal bloating can be cured permanently without removing these gallstones from the liver.

PLEASE NOTE: PRACTITIONER SUPERVISION IS HIGHLY RECOMMENDED FOR LIVER AND GALLBLADDER CLEANSE.

Preparation:

- You can't clean the liver with living parasites in it. You won't get many stones, and you can feel quite sick. Get through the first three weeks of the parasites killing program, 3-in-1 Herbs, before attempting a liver cleanse. If you are on the maintenance program, do a high-dose program the week before.

- Completing the kidney rinse before cleansing the liver is also highly recommended. You want your kidney, bladder, and urinary tract in top working condition so it can efficiently remove any undesirable substances incidentally absorbed from the intestine as the bile is being excreted (only if advised by your practitioner).

- Do any dental work first if possible. Your mouth should be metal-free and bacteria-free (cavities cleaned). A toxic mouth can put a heavy load on the liver, burdening it immediately after cleansing. Eliminate that problem first for results (only if advised by your practitioner).

- There are 10 drops of "peroxy" (35% food-grade hydrogen peroxide) in the cleanse recipe to kill bacteria and viruses as they come out of the bile ducts, also 10 drops of 3-in-1 Herbs, to kill any remaining parasites. These drops could make you feel quite ill by themselves, unless you work your way up to this dose ahead of time.

- Take one drop of "peroxy" in a beverage with each of your three meals in a day. The type of beverage does not matter; drink it throughout the meal. The purpose is to mix the peroxy thoroughly with your food. When the peroxy contacts bacteria, it fizzes, giving a sensation of nausea. If you feel sick, stay at the dosage, or less, until you feel better. The next day increase to two drops with each meal. Increase by one drop each day until you are taking five drops with each meal (seven for elderly or recently ill people). Stay at this level until you do the cleanse.

Liver Cleanse. Things you need

Epsom salts	4 dessert spoons
Olive oil	Half cup (light olive oil is easier to get down)
Fresh pink grapefruit	1 large or 2 small, enough to squeeze ⅔ to ¾ cups of juice
3-in-1 herbs	10 drops
Peroxy	10 drops
Ornithine	To aid sleep (ask your practitioner for instructions)
Large plastic straw	To help drink portions
Glass jar with lid	

Choose a day like Saturday for the cleanse, since you will be able to rest the next day.

Take no medicines, vitamins, or pills that you can do without; they can prevent success. Stop the parasite program and kidney herbs the day before too.

Eat a non-fat breakfast and lunch, such as cooked cereal with fruit, fruit juice, bread and honey (no butter or milk), baked potato, or other vegetables with salt only.

2pm. Do not eat or drink after 2 o'clock.

Get your Epsom salts ready. Mix 4 dessert spoons in 3 cups of water and pour this into a jar. This makes four servings, ¾ cup each. Set the jar in the refrigerator to get ice-cold (this is for convenience and taste only).

6pm. Drink one serving (¾) of the ice-cold Epsom salts. If you did not prepare this ahead of time, mix 1 dessert spoon in ¾ cup water now.

You may add ⅛ tsp vitamin C powder to improve the taste. You may also drink a few mouthfuls of water to rinse your mouth.

Get the olive oil and grapefruit out to warm up.

8pm. Repeat by drinking another ¾ cup of Epsom salts.

You haven't eaten since 2 o'clock, but you won't feel hungry. Get your bedtime chores done. The timing is critical for success; don't be more than ten minutes early or late.

9.45pm. Pour ½ cup (measured) olive oil into the pint jar. Squeeze the grapefruit by hand into the measuring cup. Remove pulp with a fork. You should have at least ½ cup; more (up to ¾ cup) is best. You may top it up with juice. Add this to the olive oil. Add 10 drops 3-in-1 Herbs and 10 drops of peroxy. Close the jar tightly with the lid and shake hard until watery (only fresh grapefruit does this).

Now visit the bathroom one or more times, even if it makes you late for your 10 o'clock drink. Don't be more than fifteen minutes late.

10pm. Add 1 tsp L-Ornithine powder to the above mixture. This ensures you will sleep through the night, then drink the potion you have mixed. Drinking through a large plastic straw helps it go down easier. You may use fruit juice to chase it down between sips. Take it to your bedside if you want, but drink standing up. Get it down within 5 minutes.

Lie down immediately. You might fail to get stones out if you don't. The sooner you lie down, the more stones you will get out. Be ready for bed ahead of time. Don't clean up the kitchen. As soon as the drink is down, walk to your bed and lie down flat on your back with your head up high on two pillows. Try to think about what is happening in the liver. Try to keep perfectly still for at least 20 minutes. You may feel a train of stones travelling along the bile ducts like marbles. There is no pain because the bile ducts are open (thanks to the Epsom salts!). Go to sleep.

Next morning: Upon waking, take your third dose of Epsom salts. If you have indigestion or nausea, wait until it has gone before drinking the Epsom salts. You may go back to bed. Don't take this portion before 6am

2 hours later: Take your fourth (the last) dose of Epsom salts. Drink ¾ cup of the mixture. You may go to bed.

After 2 more hours: You may eat. Start with fruit juice. Half an hour later, eat fruit. One hour later, you may eat regular food, but keep it light. By supper, you should feel recovered.

How well did you do it? Expect diarrhoea in the morning. Look to see what comes out: it is important you can report the results to your practitioner. Look for the green kind since they are genuine gallstones, not food residue since they can also be a brown colour. Only bile from the liver is pea green. The bowel movement sinks, but gallstones float because of the cholesterol inside. Count them roughly, whether tan or green.

You will need a total 2000 stones before the liver is clean enough to rid you of allergies or knee pains or upper back pains permanently. The first cleanse may rid you of them for a few days, but as the stones from the rear travel forward, they give you the same symptoms again. You may repeat cleanse at four-week intervals. Never cleanse when you are ill, eg colds or flus, etc.

Sometimes the bile ducts are full of cholesterol crystals that did not form into round stones. They appear as "chaff" floating on the top of the toilet bowl water. They may be tan coloured, harbouring millions of tiny white crystals. Cleansing this chaff is just as important as purging stones.

How safe is the liver cleanse? It is safe. My opinion is based on over 500 cases, including many people/patients in their 70s and 80s. None went to the hospital; none even reported pain. However, it can make you feel quite ill for one or two days afterwards, although in every one of these cases the maintenance parasite program had been neglected. This is why the instructions direct you to complete the parasite kidney rinse programs first, or as instructed by your practitioner.

Congratulations!

You have taken out your gallstones without surgery. I'd like to think I have perfected this recipe, but I certainly cannot take credit for its origin. It was invented hundreds, if not thousands of years ago, so THANK YOU HERBALISTS!

Reference: Hulda Clark's book, *The Cure For All Diseases*

Acknowledgements

I would like to give acknowledgement to my patients, who have taught me so much over the years and given me the privilege of helping them on their journey to wellness.

My partner, Blade Kolby Ace, who showed me how to live with an elegance of always being kind to those closest to you and has loved me dearly.

Juliet, my granddaughter who, during her cancer journey, showed me how to let go and not hang onto pain and suffering and showed me that anything was possible.

My mother, Barbara, who brought me into this world and cared for me and shared her own cancer journey, which taught me so much.

My staff and practitioners at the Natural Healing Centre, who have done nothing but support and care for me and our patients while undertaking such a big task as writing my first book.

My book mentor and publisher, Emily Gowor! Emily guided my way through this enormous process of both writing and publishing a book which is somewhat like giving birth.

Which Doctor?

Finally, to my editor Ursula who has made my book readable. Thank you so much from the bottom of my heart.

About The Author

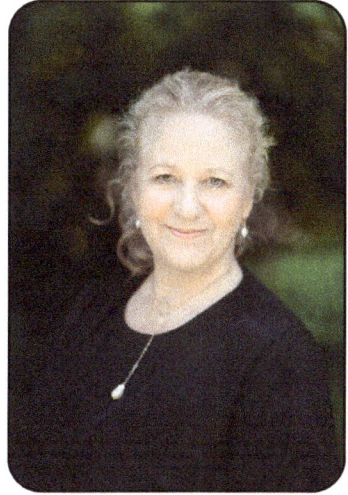

Nerida is a country girl that grew up on 1200 acres, 25 miles outside of Orange, New South Wales. As a young girl, she helped her dad at shearing time; saw baby lambs being born; helped drive cattle for 20 miles a day in the summer along the winding country roads searching for fresh grass; put her hand inside a cow to help her give birth; and, one day, shot a 303 rifle at the local country rifle club, scoring four out of five bullseyes in the target at 400 yards with her dad, one of Australia's top rifle shooters who took the Australian rifle team to win against Canada, Britain, and New Zealand.

She left home at 14 years old amidst the painful divorce of her parents, in search of happiness and good health. Years later, she ran a drug and alcohol rehab centre for 20 years, on a voluntary basis, to give back to her community and used her skills to help hundreds and hundreds of students on the program get off drugs naturally and go on to live drug-free lives. This was at the same time as running three multimodality practices in and around Melbourne, as well as mentoring over 18 other Naturopaths over her career.

Nerida spent five years developing a miraculous cream called Skin Aid, which is helping many Australians with chronic skin issues.

Today, she is running her practice in Victoria near Melbourne and dedicating her spare time to writing and teaching, hence the birth of this book, *Which Doctor?*

www.ingramcontent.com/pod-product-compliance
Lightning Source LLC
Chambersburg PA
CBHW051255020426
42333CB00026B/3225